Regardless whether the current governmental decrees restricting, and even prohibiting, public worship by the church are viewed as warranted or unnecessary, all must agree that the decrees have impinged upon, if they have not forbidden altogether, the most important activity to which humans are called: the public worship of God, by the citizens of the kingdom of the Lord Jesus. All Christians, therefore, ought to consider with utmost care the message of this book, that the Christian church is duty-bound, in perfect right, to disregard and disobey the illicit orders of the civil government restricting and even forbidding the public worship of God by the entire congregation on the Lord's Day. Uncritically to yield to the decrees of the state in the matter of public worship is indefensible. "We must obey God…" This book calls the hitherto compliant churches, including the most orthodox and conservative, which presently are not worshipping God, to repentance (sorrow over past disobedience) and conversion (change of behavior). I intend to spread the book widely in the churches in which I am a member.

---The Rev. David J. Engelsma
Emeritus Professor of Dogmatics and Old Testament
Protestant Reformed Seminary in Grand Rapids, MI

Coronavirus and the Leadership

of the Christian Church:

A Sacred Trust Broken

By

Ernest Springer, III

Joel E. Yeager, MD

Daniel O'Roark, DO, FACC

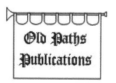

Old Paths Publications
1 Bittersweet Path
Willow Street, PA USA
...ask for the old paths... Jer. 6:16

First Edition 2020

ISBN 978-1-716-52963-4

Unless otherwise indicated, Scripture quotations are from the Authorized King James Version of The Holy Bible.

Scripture quotations labeled ESV are from the ESV® Bible (The Holy Bible, English Standard Version®), copyright © 2001 by Crossway, a publishing ministry of Good News Publishers. Used by permission. All rights reserved.

Special thanks to LuAnne D. Yeager, MD for her proof-reading and editorial work.

Old Paths Publications
would like to dedicate this book to

Dr. John F. MacArthur

&

Grace Community Church
in Sun Valley, California

for their recent faithful stand for Christian truth
and the proclamation of the Gospel of Jesus Christ

TABLE OF CONTENTS

INTRODUCTION

Ernest Springer

> "This is the day which the LORD hath made;
> we will rejoice and be glad in it."
>
> Psalm 118:24 (KJV)

"Coronavirus and the Leadership of the Christian Church: A Sacred Trust Broken". What a striking if not provocative title to address a current subject that has not only gripped the heart, mind, body, and soul of all members of the visible Church, but has also challenged the very stability and testimony of those who profess the name of Christ. As Jesus is our Lord and Savior and the very Word of Truth for all of Christian living, the desire of this book is to seek to present purity, faithfulness, and godliness in church polity and practice—from which only true peace and unity can ever be gained in Christ's Church.

With this brief introduction I want to highlight the impact of the coronavirus upon both society and the Church over the past seven months. In doing so I will also highlight the response of Church leadership as they attempted—with both compassion and good intent—to command a response by God's people to its actions and directives.

In March 2020, the alarm was sounded from our Country's highest leader of a serious danger to the citizenry of the USA and a peril faced also by the entire world. Organizations such as the World Health Organization (WHO) and the Center for Disease Control (CDC) quickly became the standard of medical statistics and guidance. In the face of death model projections expected in the millions for the USA, the names of Dr. Fauci and Dr. Birks became household companions for their supposed expertise and experience with infectious disease evaluation and recommendations. Reports of increasing infected and death numbers were being heard regularly with graph and bar chart creativity made to astonish the viewers. Daily federal press briefings about government assistance and progress to address the growing virus became a regular guest at dinner tables, followed by seemingly contentious media questions and politically charged accusations. Televised news broadcasts of Covid-19 development assumed primetime precedence nearly replacing any other local or world event. Local state governors enacted emergency disaster declarations to assume an almost martial law control with directives affecting commerce, agriculture, the financial industry, housing, commercial and retail businesses, restaurants, barbershops, educational institutions, recreational activities, and church worship gatherings just to name a few. Phrases like *stop-the-spread, flatten-the-curve, stay-at-home, essential, life-sustaining, new normal, social distancing, phases of red, yellow and green, asymptomatic,* and *my mask…your mask* mantras became some of the ever-growing novel vocabulary for the new, the different, and the strange disease being navigated. Theories of government conspiracy, international disease warfare, political maneuvering, and end-times climatic events of biblical judgment became shared dialogue through the outlets of social media, articles, viral videos, and blogs.

Throughout the above events, one common denominator obsessed the thoughts, emotions, and daily activities of the common citizen—"FEAR"! Christians were not exempt and many in the church wondered in despair. Church leaders also were not immune from the effects while at the same time burdened with the care of the flock and how best to respond. This was unchartered ground, and they found themselves grappling with the constantly changing rules and measurements of secular society to which they were looking.

The responses of church leaders varied, but almost universally churches throughout the country and much of the world reacted with one generally consistent approach: they summarily ceased public gathering for Lord's Day Worship and locked the doors of the church, forbidding their members entrance. This they said was done out of "love." All avenues of fellowship and corporate observances—such as baptism, the Lord's Supper, Sunday school, small groups, prayer meetings, Bible studies, choir, use of church library, domestic mission trips, retreats, VBS and conferences—were immediately suspended or postponed with no end date stated. Alternative forms for hearing the Word of God were provided via YouTube live-streaming broadcasts, website audio, etc. In the interim, group Bible studies and prayer meetings were conducted via telephone conference call and PC video

Zoom meetings. Many churches' ministers, elders, and deacons went above and beyond the call of duty in reaching out by telephone to their dispersed flock, seeking ways to minister to the members of the church with all means at their disposal—and doing so with all sincerity. That was to be commended as well as expected. But when would the members be able to return? These weighty decisions surely occupied the prayers and hearty debate between church leaders. All the while they received communication and concerns from the flock via email, letters, and phone calls expressing requests for return on one end and desire for continued closure on the other. This resulted in a seeming tug-of-war with potential for loss of peace and unity and a divided church.

While reentry into the building and sanctuary of the church occurred at differing times (with some still not meeting publicly even to this day), the churches set limits on the number of those who could occupy the sanctuary at one time, requiring members to register for the available seats through a website used for purchasing event tickets. How creative! They removed Bibles and hymnals from the pews, roped off every other pew for distancing, discontinued the passing of collection plates, used prepackaged elements for the Lord's Supper, wiped down pews between services, and controlled entrance and departure with ushering protocols. Many of these new routines in the church followed very closely the CDC and WHO recommendations. However, many complied with state government orders, with churches not reopening their doors until stay-at-home orders were relaxed. Even in states where religious institutions were exempt from these government orders, the pattern of agreement was almost identical. Was this coincidental or intentional?

But the difficulty of reassembling for worship was only exacerbated when church leadership, after consultation with physicians (not all of them in agreement), mandated the wearing of masks for all services and while in the church building. This requirement only heightened the concerns of those who felt that wearing a mask infringed upon their Christian liberty. Again, our leaders responded with a pattern of compliance, sticking with the recommendation of agency experts and government directives. Church leaders bought into the assumption that the seemingly healthy member in attendance might be an asymptomatic carrier. This mandate for masking in general implied that the healthy member may, in fact, be an unknown disease-walking-death-sentence to another member—yet without proof or evidence. (Some might consider this assumption to be bearing false witness.) Leadership may have seen the requirement for masking as something indifferent as regards doctrine and holy living and therefore to be legitimately imposed and tolerated. However, those who rejected the wearing of masks did so for more than simply inconvenience. As stated earlier, fear had gripped all people, resulting in even some Christians losing sight of and trust in the sovereignty of God. Hence, obligating the church member to wear a mask contributed to this fear, and that constraint became a moral issue and spiritual impediment upon a proper Christian walk and life in the church. This extra-biblical burden created upset and unrest for the believer.

In subsequent weeks, masks and face-shields were recommended but no longer required, or were mandated for specific service times, but not all services, or for specific portions of the sanctuary only, or while walking in hallways. Worship services took on the form of a virtual masknastics! Throughout this changing agenda, the requirements have taken on an equivocating seesaw swinging from Sunday to Sunday, with confused mask-on, mask-off maneuvering during worship, both in the pulpit and the pew, which if not for the solemnity of worship, would almost appear comical. However, reverence, praise, and glorifying God demands an environment free from distraction and wandering thoughts.

Finally, while some churches made known their reasons and rationale for their decisions and requirements, not all did—or at least did not do so until long into the lock-down or re-opening process. Even then the explanations that were given were sometimes only verbal, perhaps written later, and often only an explanation from a health perspective and a voiced commitment to the community. There was far too little guidance based on Biblically defined positions. There was no honest transparency if concerns surrounded insurance liability and potential monetary dangers. Questions and concerns from members to church leadership went for weeks and even months without personal reply. Some churches even accepted government offered CARES Act money which, by doing so, allows for government influence in the affairs of the church—because strings are always attached. (Might one of those strings be cooperation with the state's government contact tracing initiative?) Some churches are asking for specific information about members and their families as to who might be sick and for how long. Verbiage varies, but it goes something like this: "*Please do not come if you have Covid-19 symptoms, and please let us know if you or a household member develop symptoms or receive a positive diagnosis within 14 days of your attendance since this means you could have unknowingly been infectious.*" Was this information remaining private within the church, or was it to be available should a government request be made for it?

This begs the following questions. What can be said to all of this except, however tumultuous the times and uncertain the ends, was this an area of the Christian walk and life something to which the Scriptures did not address? Was Almighty God who created all that exists, who ordains all that comes to pass, and who by His providential acts upholds all things by His Sovereign will, unable to provide Spirit-directed guidance and instruction from the inspired, inerrant, and infallible Word of God?

How then should the Shepherds of the Church lead amidst all of this chaos? Reflect upon the timeless declarations of God in 2 Timothy 3:16-17 that "*all scripture is given by inspiration of God, and is profitable for doctrine, for reproof, for correction, for instruction in righteousness, that the man of God may be perfect, thoroughly furnished unto all good works.*"

Where do Ruling and Teaching Elders find their principles for governance? Consider their subscriptive vows to the Standards of the church, and read what is found in the 1647 Westminster Confession of Faith (WCF), Chapter 1:6 which states,

> *The whole counsel of God concerning all things necessary for his own glory, man's salvation, faith and life, is either expressly set down in Scripture, or by good and necessary consequence may be deduced from Scripture: unto which nothing at any time is to be added, whether by new revelations of the Spirit, or traditions of men. Nevertheless, we acknowledge the inward illumination of the Spirit of God to be necessary for the saving understanding of such things as are revealed in the Word: and that there are some circumstances concerning the worship of God, and government of the church, common to human actions and societies, which are to be ordered by the light of nature, and Christian prudence, according to the general rules of the Word, which are always to be observed.* [1]

---

[1] The Westminster Standards of the Presbyterian Church, which is the church of the writers, will be the main source quoted in the chapters of this book. However, many denominations maintain Standards in the form of Confessions. Below is an example of evangelical unity of doctrine on this subject agreeable to most churches:

Belgic Confession – 1561 (Reformed)

We believe that those Holy Scriptures fully contain the will of God, and that whatsoever man ought to believe, unto salvation, is sufficiently taught therein...it is unlawful for any one, though an apostle, to teach otherwise than we are now taught in the Holy Scriptures: nay, though it were an angel from heaven, as the apostle Paul saith. For, since it is forbidden, to add unto or take away anything from the word of God, it doth thereby evidently appear, that the doctrine thereof is most perfect and complete in all respects. (Art 7)

The 39 Articles of Religions – 1562 (Anglican)

Holy Scripture containeth all things necessary to salvation: so that whatsoever is not read therein, nor may be proved thereby, is not to be required of any man, that it should be

16

believed as an article of the Faith, or be thought requisite or necessary to salvation. In the name of the holy Scripture, we do understand those Canonical books of the Old and New Testament, of whose authority was never any doubt in the Church. (Art 6)

Mennonite Confession of Faith – 1963 (Mennonite)

We believe that the God of creation and redemption has revealed Himself and His will for men in the Holy Scriptures, and supremely and finally in His incarnate Son, the Lord Jesus Christ. God's purpose in this revelation is the salvation of all men... We believe that all Scripture is given by the inspiration of God, that men moved by the Holy Spirit spoke from God. We accept the Scriptures as the authoritative Word of God, and through the Holy Spirit as the infallible Guide to lead men to faith in Christ and to guide them in the life of Christian discipleship. (Art 2)

Baptist Faith & Message – 1963 (Southern Baptist)

The Holy Bible was written by men divinely inspired and is the record of God's revelation of Himself to man. It is a perfect treasure of divine instruction. It has God for its author, salvation for its end, and truth, without any mixture of error, for its matter. It reveals the principles by which God judges us; and therefore is, and will remain to the end of the world, the true center of Christian union, and the supreme standard by which all human conduct, creeds, and religious opinions should be tried. The criterion by which the Bible is to be interpreted is Jesus Christ. (Art 1)

Formula of Concord – 1577 (Lutheran)

We believe, teach, and confess that the sole rule and standard according to which all dogmas together with [all] teachers should be estimated and judged are the prophetic and apostolic Scriptures of the Old and of the New Testament alone, as it is written Ps. 119:105: Thy Word is a lamp unto my feet and a light unto my path. And St. Paul: Though an angel from heaven preach any other gospel unto you, let him be accursed, Gal 1:8. (Summary)

Articles of Religion – 1783 (Methodist)

The Holy Scripture containeth all things necessary to salvation; so that whatsoever is not read therein, nor may be proved thereby, is not to be required of any man that it should be believed as an article of faith, or be thought requisite or necessary to salvation. In the name of the Holy Scripture we do understand those canonical books of the Old and New Testaments of whose authority was never any doubt in the church. (Art 4)

Within the scope of the following chapters we will see how the Scriptures, the Confessions and Catechisms[2], church history, medical science, and governmental protection all have their respective place and benefit, lending to our wise consideration in this extraordinary time in the life of Christ's Church. Nevertheless, the operative priority must first be given to Biblical evaluation and a sacred response for faith and life that both honors our Lord and obeys His commands.

The writers of this work desire that it serves as a primer and guide for the future of the Christian Church. It is our prayerful hope that Church leadership will take this to heart as coming from brethren who offer respect and honor for the serious undertaking of shepherding the flock entrusted to them by God. It is a task with great responsibility and accountability and one where faithfulness to the Word of God is requisite, no matter what the difficulty, no matter how tenuous the outcome, and least of all, no matter the sacrifice for obedience to our Creator and Redeemer!

This therefore is why our Lord established the God-instituted Elder role with both commendation and warning. 1 Timothy 5:17 states, *"Let the elders that rule well be counted worthy of double honour, especially they who labour in the word and doctrine."* But what double portion has been warranted, when you see the plain reality of

---

[2] Confessions, Catechisms, and Statements of Faith are commonplace across many denominations and have served the church throughout its history in maintaining Biblical doctrine and practice. Nevertheless, at all times it is to be understood that while reasonably faithful and agreeable to the Bible, the Standards are not inspired, inerrant, nor infallible, and are fully subordinate to the Holy Scriptures.

unfaithfulness and disobedience? James 3:1 states, "*My brethren, be not many masters, knowing that we shall receive the greater condemnation.*" When they who are entrusted by God and by their vows to shepherd the sheep of Christ's Church have sadly failed, is the flock being complicit if they hold their peace and stay silent, or do they sound the trumpet and warn of the danger?

In the face of the varied and ever-changing directives of church leaders, peace and unity has become a casualty of invention. Without purity in doctrine and practice, division in the church will occur and has occurred. Calling attention to this error in the interest of pure doctrine and the truth of God's Word can in no way be seen as divisive, because one cannot divide that which has already been divided. To suggest otherwise is an imprudent overlooking of responsibility. To accuse those who raise concern and seek faithfulness is to criticize by intemperance and excuse first causes of the division.

In writing this book, I am blessed to be joined by two other contributors. Both are accomplished men of God whose medical vocations as physicians, along with a much studied and practical understanding of the coronavirus, remain subservient to their Savior's calling to the Office of Believer.

The first is Joel E. Yeager, MD, MA (counseling). He and his wife LuAnne D. Yeager, MD founded and operate Heritage Family Health, PC, just outside Schaefferstown, Pennsylvania. He is a Diplomate of the American Board of Family Medicine and a contributor to the Second Opinion Project. He is also the author of

Transforming Healthcare Together: Restoring the Covenant of Trust, published in 2018.

The second is Daniel O'Roark, DO, FACC, of the Ballad CVA Heart Institute in Johnson City, Tennessee. He is a Diplomate of the American Osteopathic Board of Internal Medicine/Cardiology and a Diplomate of the Certification Board of Nuclear Cardiology. He is also a Diplomate of the National Board of Echocardiography and serves as a Fellow of the American College of Cardiology.

All three writers are Presbyterians and hold to the Reformed Faith with a world and life view of God who transcends the sphere of all creation and culture. One of the writers has served as a Ruling Elder in the Orthodox Presbyterian Church (OPC) and knows the challenges of shepherding the spiritual necessities of a congregation. Another has served as a Deacon in the Presbyterian Church in America (PCA) and is well acquainted with the temporal needs of the members of a church as well as those who are resident in nursing homes. One of them has prior experience in lay-preaching. All the writers have used their skills to teach and lecture within churches, Sunday Schools, and Bible studies. Most importantly, all three believe the Word of God is preeminent for all of life and hold forth Christ as Lord of the Church and King of this world.

Chapter One, entitled "*Ecclesiásticus Interrúptio*[3] *or Why has the Church Cancelled Biblical Worship?*" is written by Ernest Springer. In

---

[3] Literally in English, "Ecclesiastical Break."

this opening chapter, the author presents a most serious subject—that of closing the House of God due to the coronavirus. It will analyze whether those in the Evangelical and Reformed community who did so were standing upon sound principles. While discoursing upon the matter of cessation of the public gathering of God's people for Lord's Day worship, the author will address a position largely focused on human consideration, convenience, and cooperation, while missing direct and clear Biblical support. It shall be affirmed that Christians should be guided by the Scriptures in all of faith and life, and that Reformed and Presbyterian believers want to be directed and governed by the Standards the Church professes to follow. Yet this chapter will also admit that neither seems to have been faithfully employed in the cessation of public worship activity, which has left the flock of Christ's Church with the feeling that they are not being shepherded and guided, but rather corralled and caged. This is a strange irony where the sheep of the Church are found pleading with their shepherds in defense of public gathering for worship in God's House!

Chapter Two, entitled *"Covid-19 Facts and Myths,"* is written by Dr. Yeager. This chapter explores three medical facts (far more prevalent and far less fatal; comorbidities are key to understanding the disease; and it's not new) and two medical myths (masks are effective and social distancing prevents asymptomatic spread) regarding Covid-19. These are crucial to understanding the misplaced response of church and society.

Chapter Three, entitled "*Covid 19, Fear and the Word of God,*" is written by Dr. O'Roark. In this chapter the author begins by distinguishing Godly (filial) fear from ungodly and sinful dread and anxiety (servile) fear. He then proceeds to demonstrate that much of the church's response to the Covid-19 pandemic is rooted in the latter.

Chapter Four, entitled "*The Necessity and Vital Importance of Jurisdictionalism (Sphere Sovereignty) to Christian and Societal Liberty: The Biblical Limitations of Civil and Ecclesiastical Power,*" is also written by Dr. O'Roark. In this chapter, the author defines and reviews the biblical and confessional basis for sphere sovereignty, its impact on Christian and societal liberty, its application to the Covid-19 narrative, and the highly adverse consequences that arise when Jurisdictionalism is abused.

Chapter Five, entitled "*A Cure Worse than the Disease,*" is written by Dr. Yeager. This chapter explores four iatrogenicides (something caused by humans rather than disease): *medical* in the form of a professional betrayal and push for a vaccine; *emotional* in the psychological problems reinforced by the unbiblical "social distancing;" *economic* in the global repercussive effects of the lockdown; and *spiritual* in the "slippery slope" we've started to descend.

In the Conclusion, all three writers will suggest a right and biblical direction for men of God who have been called as both Ruling and Teaching Elders. It will also offer a gracious encouragement to Pastors and Elders who by seeking purity will thereby affect true peace and unity.

I have set out to produce this book with the intent, purpose, and motivation of any other publishing effort previously undertaken. Old Paths Publications was established as a ministry for the cause of Christ and His Church. We seek to offer timely titles for the purpose of edification and instruction. In our day, where true Christianity is increasingly under attack, Old Paths Publications endeavors to bring together a united and confessional Reformed and Presbyterian thought through the publishing of gospel truths given to us by the Spirit of God through His faithful elect, as they saw the fast approaching storm of apostasy. Many of our published works are from the time-honored legends of the past. Occasionally, however, a modern crisis requires contemporary analysis and response. In doing so, it is my hope and prayer that we may be of service to you, that our books might ring true to the Word of God, and that the Lord Jesus Christ might be exalted by all for His own glory.

Finally, the writers present this book for the glory of our blessed Redeemer who has overcome suffering, disease, death, and the grave through His sovereign predestinating grace. And as debtors of gratitude, trusting in God's Word which is sufficient for all of life and faith, our writing is given in Jesus' name and for His eternal praise. Amen.

Ernest Springer, III
Founder & Trustee
Old Paths Publications, Inc.
October 2020

CHAPTER 1

Ecclesiásticus Interrúptio

Or

Why Has the Church Cancelled Biblical Worship?

Ernest Springer

Scripture and Church Standards

> "Praise ye the LORD.
> Praise God in his sanctuary:
> praise him in the firmament of his power."
> Psalm 150:1 (KJV)

Let us first ask a most important question. What is worship? Simply stated, worship is our response to God's revelation of His glory. In the corporate, visible body, specific worship is done in God's special presence, through the reading and especially the preaching of the Word. The Word reveals God's glory, and when confronted with God's glory, we must worship. Moses requested to be shown God's glory; his request was answered, and at once Moses worshiped (cf. Exodus 33:18; 34:5-7). Joshua also worshiped when confronted by the captain of the host of the Lord—none other than the pre-incarnate Christ (cf. Joshua 5:14). Worship is essential for the Christian, and the Scripture is essential in our understanding of worship. For therein we know the glory of God, and recognize, in the answer to question #1 of the Westminster Shorter Catechism (WSC) that,

> Man's chief end is to glorify God, and to enjoy him forever.

Second, what principles regulate our worship? Again, referring to the WSC in its answer to question #2,

> The Word of God, which is contained in the Scriptures of the Old and New Testaments, is the only rule to direct us how we may glorify and enjoy him.

This has come to be known as the *Regulative Principle of Worship*,[1] a principle abundantly presented in the Scriptures (Genesis 4:3-7; Exodus 20:4-6; 25:40; Leviticus 10:1-3; Deuteronomy 4:2; 12:32; I Samuel 13:11ff; I Kings 12:32-33; I Chronicles 15:13; II Chronicles 26:16; Jeremiah 7:31; Matthew 15:9; 28:19-20; John 4:22-24; Acts 17:23-25; Colossians 2:18-23). It teaches that we are to worship God

---

[1] This principle is rooted in the concept that God is jealous for His worship. Whereas He is perfectly holy and righteous, we even as redeemed are yet tainted in our flesh, with indwelling sin, and unable to presume upon the Lord with our own ideas and will-worship. This humble submission is distinguished from those who would claim that in the worship of God, whatever is not forbidden in the Word is allowed. Such an approach opens the door for all kinds of abuses and man-centered invention (i.e. liturgical dance, super bowl services) that dishonor our Savior.

only in ways He commands in His Word. We are not to insert into the worship service any elements which are the fabrications and inventions of man. God is honored only when we worship Him according to means set forth in His Word (either by direct commandment, Biblical example, or logical implication), and when we do not add to or take away from anything set forth therein. The Westminster Confession of Faith (WCF) in Chapter 21 (*Of Religious Worship and the Sabbath Day*) Section 1, echoes this biblical principle when it states,

> But the acceptable way of worshiping the true God is instituted by himself, and so limited by his own revealed will, that he may not be worshiped according to the imaginations and devices of men, or the suggestions of Satan, under any visible representation, or any other way not prescribed in the Holy Scripture.

That is the historical Reformed and Presbyterian position and can be seen clearly in many Reformed confessions and catechisms.

Third, when and where does the Bible instruct us to worship? The Scripture's Fourth Commandment and the Standards of the Church, expounding that command, both instruct us as to the day we are to worship, which is the New Testament Sabbath or Lord's Day. From the Old Testament, God's Fourth Commandment to *"Remember the sabbath day, to keep it holy,"* is echoed in Leviticus 19:30, *"Ye shall keep my sabbaths, and reverence my sanctuary: I am the Lord."* Here we are directed to keep the Sabbath in the Sanctuary, or the place of worship gathering where God meets His people. Also in Isaiah 58:13-

14, we read, *"If thou turn away thy foot from the sabbath, from doing thy pleasure on my holy day; and call the sabbath a delight, the holy of the Lord, honourable; and shalt honour him, not doing thine own ways, nor finding thine own pleasure, nor speaking thine own words: Then shalt thou delight thyself in the Lord...for the mouth of the Lord hath spoken it."* Man's own ways individually or collectively by church leadership is dishonorable and displeasing to God if they are contrary to His directive for Sabbath worship. In the New Testament, because of our redemption through the risen Savior, the Sabbath is the figure of the true spiritual rest we find as believers. But it is also a very real and certain day of the week in which we worship perpetually looking forward to that eternal rest in Christ Jesus, for as Hebrews 4:9 teaches, *"There remaineth therefore a rest to the people of God"* or *"a keeping of a Sabbath."*[2]

Moreover, looking at the Standards of the church which present the truth of Scripture, we can straightforwardly recognize the Westminster Divines' teaching that obedience to the Fourth Commandment is compromised by eliminating a public gathering required by Scripture. How is this so? By the word *public*. The 17th Century Westminster Larger Catechism (WLC) knew no other corporate gathering but that which was the in-person gathering of the saints:

Q117: How is the sabbath or the Lord's day to be sanctified?

A117: The sabbath or Lord's day is to be sanctified by a holy resting all the day... and making it our delight to spend the whole time...in the **public** and private exercises of **God's**

---

[2] KJV marginal translation. The original Greek is *sabbatismos*.

worship... [emphasis added] Isa. 66:23; Luke 4:16; Acts 20:7; I Cor. 16:1-2.

Clearly there is a distinction between private, family, and public or corporate worship. As stated at the beginning of this chapter, in God's special presence, specific corporate worship is conducted by the visible covenant people of God assembled publically as one body, and in one place, in reverence and praise to the Savior Jesus Christ. That this was the Biblical pattern exemplified in the Scripture is seen unmistakably. Consider the physical coming together as in 1 Corinthians 14:6, *"How is it then, brethren?* **when ye come together**...*"* [emphasis added]. And again in 1 Corinthians 11:20, *"When ye come together therefore* **into one place**...*"* [emphasis added]. Obviously, even Hebrews 10:25 has somewhat of implied application to this gathering publicly which is surely not to be neglected. The nature of these assemblies was physical and geographical in a joint location.

Most would claim these are extraordinary times requiring cessation of public gatherings, but I argue that the biblical times from when these passages were written were also extraordinary in different ways—mostly via persecution from Jews and Romans and often death—yet they gathered on the Lord's Day nonetheless (cf. many passages in the book of Acts)! But again, the Confession speaks to this as well in WCF 21:6,

> ...**public** assemblies (i.e. corporate worship), which are **not carelessly or willfully to be neglected, or forsaken,** when

God, by his Word or providence, calleth thereunto [emphasis added].

God has called us to worship corporately and publicly and nothing of this virus has providentially hindered us from being in the meeting house and sanctuary. Christ speaks in Matthew 23:37 saying "*how often would I have gathered thy children together, even as a hen gathereth her chickens under her wings, and ye would not!*" It was not God nor His Word and Providence that have hindered our meeting together for public worship!

God's mandate for weekly public Sabbath worship is not something to be trifled with or relegated to a position of lesser significance. Observing the Lord's Day in worship is no gray area or some matter of *adiaphora* (a thing indifferent). It is not simply the inconsequential matters of liberty for setting the time, length, or location of worship, understood as,

> circumstances concerning the worship of God, and government of the church, **common to human actions and societies** (WCF 1:6, emphasis added).

Rather it is the very act of choosing to follow the command to worship—the nature of which is the core essence of shepherding and gathering the sheep in fellowship to the praise of His glorious Grace, not the separation and scattering of the flock! Its unique and special nature of visible and collective communing with the risen Savior openly demonstrates the distinction and contrast from the common activities and formalities of the entrenched human life and culture separate from God and that worships itself. I would submit that the closure is to the spiritual detriment of the flock, the loss of true fellowship, and a means of Grace that is clearly not what is intended by our Lord.

Church leadership quickly closed their church buildings, effectively locking the people out of God's house. Through their enacted directives that pejoratively might be called a "stay-away-from-church" position (for that was both the desire and reality of their actions), an uncertain and nebulous parenthesis was introduced absent any studied Scriptural warrant. What then was the inducement for this radical departure from the norm of biblical practice? I will cite some areas offered as explanation for this position of cessation. While this analysis is not intended to be an exhaustive dissertation, writing on related aspects will be addressed more copiously in the chapters to follow. However, it is important to note that admittedly, their reasoned emphasis appeared to have stimuli of external concerns that were peripheral to the orderly governing of the church's worship by,

> The whole counsel of God concerning all things necessary for his own glory, man's salvation, faith and life, [which] is either **expressly set down in Scripture**, or by good and necessary consequence **may be deduced from Scripture**: unto which nothing at any time is to be added (WCF 1:6, emphasis added).

In some ways the rush to action was more a cart-before-the-horse scenario, whereby consideration and development of their alleged justification for closing should have preceded the action taken.

One rationale put forth is that we are subject to those God has placed in authority and are to obey them in all things lawful, not contrary to the Bible. That is true, but clearly the government *has* directed us to neglect the public worship of God and do something that is contrary to Scripture. However, I think it begs the question, what *has* the government directed us to do? The issue of a federal or state agency enacting directives to include church compliance regarding its worship is an authority that God has never entrusted to the magistrate. For them to do so is to misappropriate and usurp the sole rights of the Church and King Jesus. In fact, religious institutions in some states like the Commonwealth of Pennsylvania (PA), are and always have been protected by the Constitution of PA, and are specifically exempted from the closure or stay-at-home guidelines—always classifying them as essential and life-sustaining. Therefore, how the PA government feels is not relevant to how, where, or when we worship God. Yet PA churches, either intentionally or indirectly, patterned their closures in seeming lockstep to government guidelines.

However, not all states are alike, and some have directly mandated restrictions and even closures, with non-compliance punishable by fines and imprisonment. I would be remiss if I did not commend with appreciation the valiant fight by Dr. John MacArthur and Grace Community Church in Sun Valley, California for their recent faithful stand for Christian truth and the proclamation of the Gospel of Jesus Christ. They have chosen to defy the edicts of the over-reaching California government that has attempted to and ordered the church to shut down. They insist they will "have church" and that is what they have repeatedly done—all while under attack and duress from government and abandonment by friends and fellow laborers in the ministry. There are pastors who heretofore have spoken very highly of MacArthur yet today are silent, not even offering his situation in prayer before congregations. Only crickets.

Rejection and opposition to a government that oversteps its authority and threatens, shames, or harasses the Church requires courage, strength, grace, and a constant looking to God's Word through prayer. *It is very easy to make declaration in a church that we uphold the Scripture and are governed by our Standards, but when tested and tried, church leadership seems to have placed both to the back of the line in its decisioning process in favor of societal requirement and influence.* It begs the question as to how well church leadership would stand against a real governmental threat to our free and Biblical exercise of worship, like building shutdown, arrests, fines, etc. All of this for the "public good," yet how long till the government and society determine Christianity is a threat to the "public good"? Many already do. Reformation times saw people lose everything, even going to the stake for their profession and practice.

Another attempt to justify the closure of the church was by comparing it to having a gas leak in the church facility whereby imminent death may occur. Yet this example is far different than this virus issue. Some compared it to a hurricane or blizzard, where the issue of having public worship becomes a matter of Elder rule—specifically whether or not the Elders can attend to lead the worship, "piloting the ship" so to speak, for any and all who by their own choice decide to brave the elements and attend. Again, this scenario differs from the Covid-19 pandemic in that the Elders were not prevented from attending church due to this virus, neither was there an imminent nor proven expectation of infection. But in general, these comparisons are unforeseen *"acts of God"* that providentially occur outside of our control.

One of the reasons prohibiting the assembling of God's people that incorporated a biblical concept of sickness and uncleanness was in demonstrating that certain activities evidenced apparent alteration in the normal functioning of God's house. They presented the laws for quarantine as excuse for prohibiting assembly as a result of having been near a dead person or someone with leprosy. At first glance one might assume there to be a relationship, yet while not mutually exclusive from today's coronavirus, in application the concept is not even remotely the same. Certainly, if one is known to be sick, or even known to have been in compromising situations of sickness, that could somewhat relate to the leprosy, and that person should remain apart until well again. However, *the laws of the Old Testament did not require the closing of God's house,* and therein lies the rub. *You do not quarantine the healthy, only the sick.* But church leadership effectively threw away the baby with the bath water.

It seems that the mainstay upon which most churches are standing upon is genuine care, concern, and love for neighbor. We hear this almost *ad nauseam* (repeated so often that it has become tiresome). Most churches leadership's emphasis is on the second greatest commandment (to man), yet they are giving that priority over the first greatest commandment (to God) and with it, the first table of God's law (which includes the Fourth Commandment to remember the Sabbath). Actually, it is not an either-or, but by attempting to honor both together with priority to the first, we do not neglect nor do violence to the intent of love in the second. They are not mutually exclusive, but a complementary and necessary combination of obedience employed together. Public gathering for worship without the fellowship of the saints, or fellowship of the saints without public gathering for worship makes no sense and is somewhat of a *non sequitur* (a conclusion or statement that does not logically follow from the previous argument or statement). Scripture does not teach the contrary. In his article *"Coronavirus and the Church: Compliant, or Uncreative?"* in *reformation21*, Terry Johnson, Senior Pastor of Independent Presbyterian Church, in Savanah, Georgia, wrote back in early April 2020, that it has virtually, become a cliché to say that we are loving our neighbors by closing our public services.[3]

But this is a great incongruity if not absurdity. Johnson continues,

> Do our neighbors not need the prayers of the gathered church? Do our members not need the strength and refuge that the church's public services provide during unsettling times?[4]

How does the church's position and practice of "love" square with the Bible? What does the Scripture have to say about love for God and love for man?

First, in the key verse, the <u>love of God is spoken with so much more import and emphasis</u> in contrast to love of man.

> **Mark 12:30-31:** [30]And thou shalt love the Lord thy God with all thy heart, and with all thy soul, and with all thy mind, and with all thy strength: this is the first commandment. [31]And the second is like, namely this, Thou shalt love thy neighbour as thyself...

Second, the overwhelming and majority of verses in the Bible have emphasis on God and to a lesser degree on man. Even more

---

[3] Johnson, https://www.reformation21.org/blog/coronavirus-and-the-church-compliant-or-uncreative?fbclid=IwAR3ar6lgbNVGTvdCHO3ZkaC4rSVlWfx2uDfOhV_4ybvJg-TUU9JSRW6IRD_4, accessed 9/9/2020.

[4] Ibid.

striking is that the Scripture speaks of <u>our love of God</u> repeatedly in the same verses, <u>in conjunction with our obedience to His commands</u>.

> **Deuteronomy 7:9:** Know therefore that the Lord thy God, he is God, the faithful God, which keepeth covenant and mercy with them that love him and keep his commandments to a thousand generations.

> **Deuteronomy 10:12-13:** [12]And now, Israel, what doth the Lord thy God require of thee, but to fear the Lord thy God, to walk in all his ways, and to love him, and to serve the Lord thy God with all thy heart and with all thy soul, [13]To keep the commandments of the Lord, and his statutes, which I command thee this day for thy good?

Third, they speak of the <u>keeping of these commandments as needing to be done always</u>.

> **Deuteronomy 11:1:** Therefore thou shalt love the Lord thy God, and keep his charge, and his statutes, and his judgments, and his commandments, alway.

Fourth, they speak of such <u>obedience to His commands being an evidence of that love of God and love of man</u>.

> **1 John 5:2:** By this we know that we love the children of God, when we love God, and keep his commandments.

Lastly, we are told that the <u>very definition of love of God is the keeping of His commandments</u>.

1 John 5:3: For this is the love of God, that we keep his commandments: and his commandments are not grievous.

In summary then, it is clear from the above verses that the love of God has greater significance than the love of man, it is never to be separated from obedience to His commandments, His commandments are to be kept always, the keeping of them is an evidence of our love of God and of man, and the keeping of His commandments is the very definition of love of God—which includes the full keeping of the Fourth Commandment.

While churches with sincere motives chose to place such emphasis on love of neighbor, nonetheless in their exercise of such (appealing to a minority of passages), this same Bible nowhere, and I repeat *nowhere*, affords them the authority to lessen or contravene the Biblical dictates of the Fourth Commandment and the requirement for the gathering of the public assembly of God's people in God's house. To do so is to ignore the teaching of the Bible and is disobedience to the Holy Spirit, the author of Holy Scripture.

When it comes to the disorder and confusion of our culture, our community, and the citizens surrounding us, we see that America is a society that is fearful and especially fears death—for apart from the saving work of Christ, they have no hope. Regrettably, the Church today appears to think and act too much like the world, showing the same lack of faith. Are we just weak and erring Christians, or does the church institute act like the world because that is where their heart is? Have we allowed the world to influence the Church rather than being salt and light to humanity? Are our hearts set upon those things above or are we fixated upon the creature comforts of the earth? These are penetrating questions, to be sure, but it suggests the desire for superfluity, protection, ease of obligation, a yield to medicine over Scripture, and escape from what is likely the judgment of God both upon the world and the modern Church today. That is how it all appears, albeit for love of people's health and well-being.

Church leadership made the decisions when to close and when to open in consultation with physicians, *weighing the majority and most convincing assessment of health risk* to build its narrative. *But that is problematic, as risk should not be a prelude to evaluation of how to understand the Scripture.* Rather, a biblical position and foundation must first be established in order to see how best to apply and work through that risk. However, the presumption of medical consideration seems to be the first area dealt with, then with that presupposition, if you will, determinative resolution is made. We cannot establish the catalyst of influence for decisions in the church by the opinion of doctors before the analysis and substance of Scripture. *Risk is never the primary factor upon which the scales of God's commandments should lean.* The Christian's call is to determine, *"What saith the Scripture?"* (Romans 4:3). Yet even therein we must reflect upon the limits of church leaders in the face of medical analysis because there exists an inherent spiritual right that must allow the Office of Believer to manage their own bodies and health. Church leaders should leave the decision up to the members of the church whether they want to govern themselves and their families by being present for the Worship of God. Isn't that a decision that believers in Christ and fathers as heads of household should be able to make, trusting by faith and willing to endure the Providences of a Sovereign God? Sickness and disease are remarkable reminders of the consequences of sin and God's righteous judgment. That's not exactly what you hear in the doctor's office, but it is marvelous to hear from the pulpit! Many physicians—even Christian ones—sometimes view issues of health and sickness through a different prism than one who considers ideas through the lens of Scripture.

My wife and I were members 35 years ago at Philadelphia's Tenth Presbyterian Church where the late James Montgomery Boice was minister. Dr. Boice would annually gather graduating medical school students from the Philadelphia area who were attending Tenth and before praying for them in the presence of the congregation and God, he would give them a solemn charge. This charge not only directed to them to make wise and ethical medical decisions in their practice, but being Christians, to see their vocation as being not mutually exclusive from their Christian profession and the requirements of truth found in the Scriptures and Standards of the church. How significant a church practice that counseled the young physicians to place the wisdom of God's Word above and before the knowledge of medical science!

I am reminded of Job and his sufferings, which amongst other things were certainly a matter of health (perhaps even leprosy, though we don't know that for sure or may have been scabies, both of which were a contagion to others, the latter even more so). But I am struck by Job's statement of faith in Job 23:12, *"Neither have I gone back from the commandment of his lips; I have esteemed the words of his mouth more than my necessary food."* Job's assurance in the midst of suffering led him early on, before even the worst of trials upon his health, to proclaim in Job 1:21, *"Naked came I out of my mother's womb, and naked shall I return thither: the LORD gave, and the LORD hath taken away; blessed be the name of the LORD."* His life experience is also seen in Christ's words for children of faith in Luke 12:22-32, *"...Take no thought for your life, what ye shall eat; neither for the body, what ye shall put on. The life is more than meat, and the body is more than raiment...O ye of little faith? And seek not ye what ye shall eat, or what ye shall drink, neither be ye of doubtful mind. For all these things do the nations of the world seek after...But rather seek ye the kingdom of God; and all these things shall be added unto you. Fear not, little flock; for it is your Father's good pleasure to give you the kingdom."*

Like Job, the Scriptures provide wonderful examples of how God's people, facing illness, terror, fearful trials, persecution, and all kinds of suffering, pursued the best medicine for their woes. Like Jehoshaphat (cf. 2 Chronicles 20:1-3), they sought communion with the Lord for deliverance. Like Hezekiah (cf. 2 Kings 20:1-6), they turned to God in prayer for healing. Like David, they brought their supplications before Jehovah as seen in so many of the Psalms. True believers throughout the Bible approached the Father's throne with boldness and confidence knowing that He alone is the God who will hear and who will answer and bring comfort in time of need.

Church History

> "I will praise thee, O LORD, among the people: and I will sing praises unto thee among the nations."
> Psalm 108:3 (KJV)

We have considered the requisite testimony of Holy Scripture and some brief doctrinal divinity in our Church Confessions and Catechisms. While outside of these aforementioned authorities, the history of the Church and how men of faith in practice touched upon our subject at hand, though to a lesser degree, can be very instructive for the people of God. The accounts, statements, and attitudes of whom I refer to affectionately as "old dead guys" bring a word of man, with "*God testifying of his gifts: and by it he being dead yet speaketh.*" (Hebrews 11:4). As they were theologians, pastors, teachers, and elders in the church, they often have a timeless unction from the experimental working of the Lord in their life and times, which should be heeded by Church leaders today.

The Early Church

An interesting article of argument entitled *"Christianity Has Been Handling Epidemics for 2000 Years,"*[5] was written by Lyman Stone, a research fellow at the Institute for Family Studies and an advisor at the consulting firm Demographic Intelligence. Stone has also served as a missionary in Hong Kong. Stone references two ancient plagues from the early Christian Church.

The Antonine Plague of 165 to 180 AD

This plague, also known as the Plague of Galen, was an ancient pandemic brought to the Roman Empire by troops who were returning from campaigns in the Near East. Scholars have suspected it to have been either smallpox or measles. As Stone writes,

> During plague periods in the Roman Empire, Christians made a name for themselves. Historians have suggested that the terrible Antonine Plague of the 2nd century, which might have killed off a quarter of the Roman Empire, led to the spread of Christianity, as Christians cared for the sick and offered an spiritual model whereby plagues were not the work of angry and capricious deities but the product of a broken Creation in revolt against a loving God.[6]

---

[5] Stone, https://foreignpolicy.com/2020/03/13/christianity-epidemics-2000-years-should-i-still-go-to-church-coronavirus/?fbclid=IwAR0zzwJoeaswxXltb3jVz9_imeoCY-beyf5p_PjLKSG0gh9SUYQC73oFmdkw, accessed 8/19/2020.

[6] Ibid.

The plague was named after St. Cyprian, bishop of Carthage, an early Christian writer who witnessed and provided a colorful account of this disease in his sermons. While there is some uncertainty, the nature of this plague may have been smallpox, pandemic influenza, or viral hemorrhagic fever (filoviruses) like the Ebola virus. Stone continues,

> The Plague of Cyprian helped set off the Crisis of the Third Century in the Roman world. But it did something else, too: It triggered the explosive growth of Christianity. Cyprian's sermons told Christians not to grieve for plague victims (who live in heaven), but to redouble efforts to care for the living. His fellow bishop Dionysius described how Christians, "Heedless of danger … took charge of the sick, attending to their every need."[7]

He continues saying,

> Nor was it just Christians who noted this reaction of Christians to the plague. A century later, the actively pagan Emperor Julian would complain bitterly of how "the Galileans" would care for even non-Christian sick people, while the church historian Pontianus recounts how Christians

---

[7] Ibid.

ensured that "good was done to all men, not merely to the household of faith."[8]

Before moving on to the times of the Reformers, I want to offer a longer section from Stone where he sums up what should be the understanding from the examples of the early church and why gathering together as a community of believers, even in times of pandemic, is so very important and necessary.

> This brings me to one of the more controversial elements of historic Christian plague ethics: We don't cancel church. The whole motivation of personal sacrifice to care for others, and other-regarding measures to reduce infection, presupposes the existence of a community in which we're all stakeholders. Even as we take communion from separate plates and cups to minimize risk, forgo hand-shaking or hugging, and sit at a distance from each other, we still commune.

> Some observers will view this as a kind of fanaticism: Christians are so obsessed with church-going that they'll risk epidemic disease to show up.

> But it's not that at all. The coronavirus leaves over 95 percent of its victims still breathing. But it leaves virtually every member of society afraid, anxious, isolated, alone, and wondering if anyone would even notice if they're gone. In an

---

[8] Ibid.

increasingly atomized society, the coronavirus could rapidly mutate into an epidemic of despair. Church attendance serves as a societal roll call, especially for older people: Those who don't show up should be checked on during the week. Bereft of work, school, public gatherings, sports and hobbies, or even the outside world at all, humans do poorly. We need the moral and mental support of communities to be the decent people we all aspire to be.

The Christian choice to defend the weekly gathering at church is not, then, a superstitious fancy. It's a clear-eyed, rational choice to balance trade-offs: We forgo other activities and take great pains to be as clean as possible so that we can meaningfully gather to support each other.[9]

Martin Luther & the German Lutherans

Some today have rested in solace referencing a 1527 writing from Luther entitled *"Whether One May Flee From A Deadly Plague"*[10] in which he excuses some ministers who desire to abscond from the plague. A snippet of this has been bandied about by some today,

---

[9] Ibid.

[10] Luther, Luther's Works, Vol. 43: Devotional Writings II, ed. Jaroslav Jan Pelikan, Hilton C. Oswald, and Helmut T. Lehmann, vol. 43 (Philadelphia: Fortress Press, 1999), 119–38. It is also found online at:
https://blogs.lcms.org/wp-content/uploads/2020/03/Plague-blogLW.pdf?fbclid=IwAR3XKNLo1kG5YH6VJE0LH0AVWvmYtWgh86xIOR20S1lc2S71mSL4jZZrjaA, accessed 8/19/2020.

including a series by Westminster Theological Seminary professors sitting in their armchairs. It is hailed as support for the cessation of public gathering for worship. However, some interesting facts of conscience and faith have not been forthcoming, and one must read the entire letter of Luther to a pastor during this plague.

First, Luther says nothing of suspending worship, but rather that the city had

> enough preachers[11]

and that

> spiritual services are provided for.[12]

That is noteworthy in and of itself, for there was not a wholesale abandonment of the city. In fact, Luther, Bugenhagen, and two chaplains stayed on at Wittenberg. Luther states plainly,

> Those who are engaged in a spiritual ministry such as preachers and pastors must likewise remain steadfast before the peril of death. We have a plain command from Christ, "A good shepherd lays down his life for the sheep but the hireling sees the wolf coming and flees" [John 10:11]. For when people are dying, they most need a spiritual ministry which strengthens and comforts their consciences by word and sacrament and in faith overcomes death.[13]

---

[11] Ibid.

[12] Ibid.

[13] Ibid.

It is quite curious that the Westminster Seminary professors left this out of their discussion.

Secondly, it is overwhelmingly evident that those who avoid the plague are spoken of as weak in the faith and given over to fear. Specifically, Luther calls them

weak and fearful[14]

The point then is that he no doubt says, *go ahead and flee, for such a one as you are of no value here to minister to the sick and dying.* And therein lies the rub. Let those who have closed the doors of the church today go out and **personally** minister to, pray with, and encourage those infected and dying of the coronavirus. This is their duty, and this is what Luther's letter explains. But this is hardly seen nor heard in the present crisis! Oh, but the government has restricted entry to the sick. This, however, should have been rejected by the Church and aggressively fought against, but church leaders would not.

John Calvin & the Swiss Reformed

Dr. Harry L. Reeder III, senior pastor of Briarwood Presbyterian Church in Birmingham, Alabama, has written of how John Calvin courageously faced repeated outbreaks of plague during his ministry in Geneva:

---

[14] Ibid.

During Calvin's ministry, Geneva was terrorized by the plague on five occasions. During the first outbreak, in 1542, Calvin personally led visitations into plague-infected homes. Knowing that this effort likely carried a death sentence, the city fathers intervened to stop him because of their conviction that his leadership was indispensable. The pastors continued this heroic effort under Calvin's guidance, and they recounted the joy of multiple conversions. Many pastors lost their lives in this cause. Unknown to many, Calvin privately continued his own pastoral care in Geneva and other cities where the plague raged. Calvin's pastoral heart, already evidenced by the provision of hospitals for both citizens and immigrants, was further revealed as he collected the necessary resources to establish a separate hospital for plague victims. When believers died, he preached poignant funeral homilies with passion and personal concern.[15]

From the available writings of Calvin and Geneva's Ecclesiastical Ordinances, we do not know exactly how the Geneva churches adjusted their worship services, if at all, because of the plague. The plague-infected citizens were quarantined outside the walled city in hospitals, while the Genevan churches' healthy remained inside the city behind the wall. As stated by Barry Waugh in "John Calvin & Plagues,"

---

[15] Reeder, (John Calvin: A Heart for Devotion, Doctrine, and Discipleship, ed. Burk Parsons [Lake Mary, FL: Reformation Trust, 2008], 65).

Geneva had an intermingling or fusion of church and state, which was clearly exhibited in the magistracy transgressing the spiritual ministry of the church by excluding Calvin from hospital visitation because of his importance as a Reformer.[16]

In other words, the city leaders sinned by their restricting Calvin. There was nothing in this restriction that limited Calvin from his spiritual duties in Genevan public worship; in fact, Calvin's regular regiment was to preach multiple times through the week. Despite the authority of Geneva's "city fathers" attempting restraint of Calvin, he and other ministers continued to minister to the sick. Some of them even died, knowing the risks. In addition, in this troubling time of plague, Calvin preached funeral sermons. Calvin did not preach to a dead person in a casket. He preached to the living, as he did always, and did so publicly. The elements of public gathering were deemed necessary for this ministerial service. Are today's closed churches doing the same?

Daniel Defoe & the Anglicans of London

The history of the church in times of plagues typically do not support cessation of public gathering for worship. There is an interesting and timely old book called *A Journal of the Plague Year*[17] by

---

[16] Waugh, https://www.presbyteriansofthepast.com/2020/03/22/john-calvin-plagues/, accessed 8/19/2020.

[17] Defoe, https://www.gutenberg.org/files/376/376-h/376-h.htm, accessed 8/19/2020.

Daniel Defoe which is the account of the Plague in London in 1665, a good read for our times. Consider the following from the account that shows the driving faithful determination by some to maintain their station, to stay at the post, and fulfil the obligatory service to God's people. And the people, yes, the people, came to hear the Word preached and to receive prayer for the trials that besought them.

> Besides, there were some people who, notwithstanding the danger, did not omit publicly to attend the worship of God, even in the most dangerous times; and though it is true that a great many clergymen did shut up their churches, and fled, as other people did, for the safety of their lives, yet all did not do so. Some ventured to officiate and to keep up the assemblies of the people by constant prayers, and sometimes sermons or brief exhortations to repentance and reformation, and this as long as any would come to hear them. And Dissenters did the like also, and even in the very churches where the parish ministers were either dead or fled.[18]

Can one find a more striking example of courage and correctness in the time of plague?

---

[18] Ibid.

Charles Haddon Spurgeon & the English Baptists

Moving then to another example of churches and their leaders doing what is right, we turn to The Gospel Coalition and an article by Geoff Chang entitled, *"Five Lessons from Spurgeon's Ministry in the 1854 Cholera Outbreak."*[19] Of particular interest is the second lesson which I quote below:

> #2 - Spurgeon Adjusted His Meetings But Continued Meeting
>
> The Broad Street Cholera Outbreak of 1854 occurred in August and September of that year, and its effects were felt in the weeks and months to come. The neighborhood where Spurgeon's church met was not quarantined, so they were able to continue meeting throughout those months. Interestingly, no record of the sermons Spurgeon preached during those days remain. Perhaps the outbreak forced the congregation to adjust some of their previous practices, including the transcription of sermons. Additionally, Spurgeon was likely too busy in those days to edit sermons for publication.
>
> Yet we know that the congregation continued meeting during those days, because the church's minute books contain records of congregational meetings throughout fall 1854. In those books, amid all the pastoral challenges of the

---

[19] Spurgeon, https://www.thegospelcoalition.org/article/spurgeon-ministry-cholera-outbreak/, accessed 8/19/2020.

outbreak, Spurgeon and his deacons continued to receive new members, pursue inactive members, observe the Lord's Supper, and practice all the other normal activities of a church. Not only that, but in retrospect it was particularly during this time, when news of death raged all around the city, that Spurgeon found Londoners most receptive to the gospel.

> If there ever be a time when the mind is sensitive, it is when death is abroad. I recollect, when first I came to London, how anxiously people listened to the gospel, for the cholera was raging terribly. There was little scoffing then.[20]

In other words, not only did Spurgeon gather his church amid the outbreak, but he saw in these gatherings a uniquely powerful opportunity for the gospel. In obedience, the leaders of his church worshiped with a mind's eye to the goal of evangelism. The personal delivery of the message of redemption in Christ occupied the thoughts and hearts of those to whom it had been entrusted. No such elocution requisite for exhortation can ever be successfully accomplished and with the blessing of Spirit-filled empowerment apart from God's people gathered before the pulpit!

The Message of Historical Practice for the Church Today

From all of these above examples, beginning with the Early Church, and spanning through the years of Renaissance,

---

[20] Ibid.

Reformation, Enlightenment, and the Industrial Revolution, the Church made both its witness and its presence known and felt in times of plague and distress. They did not hide. They did not put self-preservation above personal visitation and caring for the sick. Their witness of the Gospel was evident in word and deed. They willingly defied state authority and recognized their calling and duties as coming from a higher spiritual authority. Nor did they cease in meeting the needs of the community of saints, physically, emotionally, and spiritually through the gathering for worship with preaching, prayer, and praise of our great God of Peace.

In great contrast to the past, this then is the sad commentary on our modern age of the 2020 coronavirus. Midway through the lock-down of the church, a rather pungent yet truthful assessment in *Pulpit & Pen* was offered entitled, "Did Your Church Close? It's Beyond Time to Repent and Apologize." The writer, JD Hall, sounds the alarm of the lost opportunity for witness by the church and a weakened testimony of faithfulness to the Bible, saying,

> God gave churches a perfect opportunity over the last six weeks. If Christians had only been obedient to the Bible, faithful in their assembling, and steadfast in their resolve to worship, they could have been seen as the right ones all along. Instead, most churches trembled in boots and turned

out the lights right when they should have been shining the brightest.[21]

In a writing a couple months later from the American Mind entitled "The COVID Coup," Angelo Codevilla, having seen beyond the settled dust, says,

> Had this generation of church leaders simply practiced their faith, even by merely keeping silent about the ruling class's claims about the COVID-19 rather than ignorantly, submissively endorsing them, they would have preserved their intellectual and moral credit to help the general population to deal with the growing realization that they had been duped.[22]

In other words, amongst the world of disillusioned people, the credibility of the Church has been diminished if not lost altogether in the minds of some who see church leaders' support of societal panic no different than secular culture whose trust is in themselves and in government control.

---

[21] Hall, https://pulpitandpen.org/2020/04/22/did-your-church-close-its-beyond-time-to-repent-and-apologize/?fbclid=IwAR3qjKijQJaU-NOE91fej_jP8ekF9Odhy1d1Z91otNv4uw6v5_8j-ocyUNPc, accessed 8/19/2020.

[22] Codevilla, https://americanmind.org/essays/the-covid-coup/?fbclid=IwAR0sC4ZI3yBh-Kium8F6En8C8pCixIDbHt89_zzXQ3RPDNWApGWQ46j0hODE, accessed 8/20/2020.

More recently in *The Daily Signal*, David Hunter, in his article "In a Flourishing Society, Should Safety Be a Means or an End?" states,

> Education, friendship, virtue, and worship all arise from our unique identity as humans. Since God created us this way, a flourishing human life must contain each of these facets... Thus, we should protect ourselves and others, especially those most vulnerable to this disease, but these precautions must not eliminate activities that constitute a distinctly human life... As responsible, rational creatures, we should consider safety but not enthrone it as the purpose of life. Rather than ask what is safe, we should ask what is good.[23]

And worship is good! "*It is a **good** thing to give thanks unto the Lord, and to sing praises unto thy name, O Most High*" (Psalm 92:1, emphasis added). Worship is good because the God we worship is good! "*And when all the children of Israel saw how the fire came down, and the glory of the Lord upon the house, they bowed themselves with their faces to the ground upon the pavement, and **worshipped**, and praised the Lord, saying, For **he is good**; for his mercy endureth for ever*" (2 Chronicles 7:3, emphasis added).

Finally, a fervor of righteous indignation for the glory of God and His command of Lord's Day worship is seen in another article

---

[23] Hunter, https://www.dailysignal.com/2020/08/18/in-a-flourishing-society-should-safety-be-a-means-or-an-end/#disqus_thread, accessed 8/20/2020.

from *Pulpit & Pen* entitled, "ReOpen Church Sunday' Campaign Launched To Urge Mass Church Openings." Dustin Germain wrote the following:

> Rather, churches should be assembled this Sunday for their services. That's two days away. Not next week. 48 hours from now. And quite frankly, one of the very first things that most pastors should do is ensure their prepared message has a big long section where they repent and ask their churches to forgive them for being closed in the first place, for allowing fear to foment rather than being faithful…The pastors don't need to add caveats, explanations or excuses for why they closed in the first place. Rather they should admit their error, explain why it was an error, ask for forgiveness, then move forward while thanking God that the shame of their actions has led them to repentance.[24]

Consider all that has been argued in this chapter and see if truth has been spoken. I leave it to the reader to assess if the above admonishments are warranted. Not all Sessions, Consistories, or church Board members decide matters rightly all the time. After all they, just as we, are sinners saved by Grace. In fact, WCF 31:3 states,

---

[24] Germain, https://pulpitandpen.org/2020/04/24/reopen-church-sunday-campaign-launched-to-urge-mass-church-openings-on-may-3/?fbclid=IwAR1lVDEblm-poemFvF9eA2EsmqIdm666ChZvvQP38_W0_cBWpoGcpwPaNaTY, accessed 8/19/2020.

All synods or councils, since the apostles' times, whether general or particular, may err; and many have erred. Therefore they are not to be made the rule of faith, or practice; but to be used as a help in both.

We might learn by way of application from the minor prophet Haggai, where the Israelites, cowering under fear of the people, found comfort and safety in their homes. Although tending to the daily activities of life, they were met with small returns because they neglected their first duty and left the House of God in disrepair. I can't help but see a striking comparison to our age of choosing fear over faithfulness by locking down the House of Worship. They did not realize the fruitless efforts for their daily sustenance as a chastening of God. They are twice reprimanded by the Lord, and challenged in Haggai 1:5 and again in Haggai 1:7, *"Thus saith the LORD of hosts; Consider your ways,"* or more literally in the Hebrew, *"Set your heart on your ways."*

Church leaders may defensively state that they stand behind the decisions made at that time based upon the information they had at their disposal. Yet the Holy Scriptures were always available to hearts receptive to truth! We know from Jeremiah 17:9 that, *"The heart is deceitful above all things, and desperately wicked: who can know it?"* If you are a church leader, then consider in your own heart, which this writer cannot judge, if error against truth and the Savior has been made in the cessation of public worship in your church. We've looked at the words of Scripture, the witness of the Standards, and examples of the Church's history. If errors were made, then a prescription for forgiveness is vital to regain and secure purity thereby to obtain true peace and unity in the Church.

CHAPTER 2

Covid-19 Facts and Myths

Joel E. Yeager, MD

The genesis of this chapter dates to early April 2020, only several weeks after President Trump declared a national state of emergency on March 13, 2020. To be certain, none of us knew in March what we were dealing with and so caution was in order. Early on, I began to "smell a rat" and posted something on my personal Facebook page comparing Covid-19[1] with the annual influenza. I received some harsh criticism from several physicians and so I opted to delete the post, hunker down without public comment, keep our office open rather than shut, and continue to observe. We had already observed the "sickest" season in our office history from early January through mid-

---

[1] This footnote clarifies nomenclature (naming) of the virus. Note that on February 11, 2020, the International Committee on Taxonomy of Viruses named SARS-CoV-2 as *the virus* responsible for Covid-19 (*the disease*), according to this source at the WHO. It was named CoV-2 because of its genetic similarity to the coronavirus responsible for the SARS outbreak of 2003. Note also that "a close study of circulating [SARS-CoV-2] viral genomes suggests that the first infection and human-to-human spread occurred between mid-September and early December 2019," according to the AAPS May 2020 newsletter. Covid-19 is sometimes written as COVID-19 in the literature. I have chosen the former convention unless otherwise quoting.

March, *prior to* the emergency shutdown, i.e. patients were much sicker *then* than *now*.[2]

This reality prompted me to write a letter to our Pennsylvania Governor Tom Wolf on April 25th. I posted the letter to our office website and then distributed it via several social media channels. Within 36 hours our office website had received nearly 4,000 hits.[3] The letter—which is more aptly a 10-page scientific report—traveled widely throughout the community and country. Dr. Jaan Sidorov, CEO and President of the PA Clinical Network at the Pennsylvania Medical Society, called it "the best science-based critical examination of the key assumptions underlying Harrisburg's response to the coronavirus that I have seen.[4] We received multiple calls, emails, and letters from patients and non-patients expressing appreciation for having been given a voice. Some of my contributions to this booklet are a result of the research I did for the letter.

---

[2] That has remained consistently true through this writing (presently 8/29/20). Our local office spike of Covid-19 occurred in late May, peaking throughout mid to late June, and gradually tapering off through this writing. This is based on a combination of positive Covid-19 swabs and/or clinical symptoms consistent with Covid-19 treated either via phone or in person at our office.

[3] The purpose of this letter (still available on the homepage at www.heritagefamilyhealth.org) was to offer a perspective from a large primary care practice that didn't align with or support the draconian measures taken by our Governor and Health Secretary as well as to outline how shutdown was causing far greater harm than Covid-19 itself.

[4] This was in an email copied to our office dated 4/30/2020. In subsequent correspondence with Dr. Sidorov, he (an editor of a medical journal) suggested I submit it to a first-tier journal such as *JAMA* or *NEJM* and even edited it to journal form for me.

This chapter will outline three medical facts and two medical myths regarding coronavirus. I preface these with five caveats. *First, I write from a Christian worldview.*[5] This is not at all in conflict with science, for an ordered universe based upon a predictable moral law given by a Moral Lawgiver is what has given rise to the very possibility of the scientific method. C. S. Lewis wrote in the last line of his essay "Is Theology Poetry?": "I believe in Christianity as I believe that the Sun has risen, not only because I see it, but because by it I see everything else."[6]

Second, science is limited to observations about reality. We live in an era where science has become its own god, and folks subscribing to that "religion" believe that something does not exist if it isn't proven by science. In fact, there are current yard creed signs in our local community espousing a far-left political ideology; one of the lines states "I believe in science." I suspect the implication is that those who challenge a scientific narrative do not believe in science. While that could certainly be the case, that conclusion does not logically follow and is hence a *non sequitur.* I will aim to show that much of what is masquerading as science in relation to coronavirus is exactly that—a

---

[5] Yeager, Joel E. (2018). *Transforming Healthcare Together: A Model for Restoring the Covenant of Trust.* Newmanstown, PA: Heritage Imprints. I would encourage you to read Appendix 1 entitled "Why Does Worldview Matter?"

[6] Lewis, C.S. (1949, 1962, 1965, 1975, 1980). *The Weight of Glory and Other Addresses.* (W. Hooper, Ed.) New York: Simon & Schuster, p. 106.

masquerade.[7] C. S. Lewis addressed this very concept in his 1943 BBC radio talks when he said, "Do not think I am saying anything against science: I am only saying what its job is."[8] He goes on to state that "real scientists" do not usually make statements about things which are not scientific, but that "it is usually the journalists and popular novelists who have picked up a few odds and ends of half-baked science from textbooks who go in for them."[9] It sounds like he was writing about the popular media and Hollywood in 2020!

Third, I am not attempting to present a complete overview of Covid-19. There are and will be books written on this! I am responding from my own clinical experience to some specific issues as relates to church and community such as mask-wearing and social distancing. I have reason to believe that my conclusions can easily be extrapolated to most of the American population. I am also not addressing the origin of Covid-19, although it's incumbent on honest enquirers to research this.

Fourth, I am not a Covid expert. However, I am responding out of 20 years of clinical experience.[10] I have been in my profession long

---

[7] A *masquerade* is a false show or pretense and is often associated with masquerade balls where people wear masks!

[8] Lewis, C. S. (1943, 1945, 1952, 1980). *Mere Christianity.* New York: Simon & Schuster, A Touchstone Book, p. 32.

[9] Ibid.

[10] LuAnne and I have a collective 40 years of clinical experience from the time we started "storming the wards" in the year 2000 as medical students at Ninewells Hospital in Dundee, Scotland.

enough to see recommendations be turned on their heads only to swing back to the original recommendation. Sadly, our society lacks both wisdom and common sense. One thing I appreciate more with each passing year is how often those two qualities are demonstrated in my own patients. Sometimes we place far too much stock in what the "experts" say. I'm reminded of what Larry Crabb said when I was in one of his classes in the foothills of the Rockies in 1996. A troubled couple came to him for counseling and he thought to himself, *you should see an expert*. Then he realized he *was* the expert!

I was introduced to the works of Rabbi Edwin Friedman about eight years ago while doing some doctoral leadership training. Friedman was a family therapist and highly regarded leadership consultant working amongst the power brokers of Washington, DC for over 35 years. In a chapter entitled "Data Junkyards and Data Junkies," he writes about "the fallacy of expertise."

> As long as leaders—parents, healers, managers—base their confidence on how much data they have acquired, they are doomed to feeling inadequate, forever. They will never catch up.[11]

> Concerning physicians, the data deluge can distract them from focusing on the healing power contained within their own presence.[12]

---

[11] Friedman, Edwin H. (1999, 2007). *A Failure of Nerve: Leadership in the Age of the Quick Fix.* New York: Seabury Books, p. 96.

[12] Ibid, p. 101.

Daily, the media publish the latest results of some "scientific" discovery...The overall nerve-wracking effect on patients is many-fold.[13]

It is almost as though the more knowledgeable one tries to be, the more anxious one must necessarily become.[14]

While studies of pathology are useful in the treatment and prevention of disease..., there are equally great lessons to be learned from those tragedies about the tenacity of life and the capacity of members of the human race to endure and overcome.[15]

The assumption that data and technique are the keys to life is a major distortion of reality; many professionals organize their entire life around the symptoms of imbibing more of the substance...[16]

...to use a spiritual metaphor, the worship of data and technique is very simply a form of idolatry.[17]

---

[13] Ibid, pp. 103-4.

[14] Ibid, p. 105.

[15] Ibid, p. 108. This is apropos in relation to our current media's coverage of Covid, where daily counts and death rates are held ever before us *while largely ignoring* the much greater set of data of those who recover without incident.

[16] Ibid, p. 115.

[17] Ibid, p. 116. None of these quotes are to imply that Friedman thought there was no purpose in data. However, data must be subservient to a larger purpose. If he were still living, I suspect he would fiercely critique how both data and a skewed view of data has shaped society's (both church and government) response to coronavirus.

Finally, I do not take Covid-19 lightly. It is a real disease which "can cause respiratory and multi-organ failure; occasionally strikes down young, healthy individuals with terrifying speed; has overwhelmed intensive care units in some areas; and is highly contagious."[18] I had one patient die of this disease, and I feel the family's pain and loss. Patients are more than statistics. Statistics cited throughout the rest of the chapter are held in tension with the stories and faces of patients across the country. But only an honest appraisal of statistics will enable us to avoid repeating "the well-intentioned errors of our past."[19]

We begin with some medical facts before addressing medical myths regarding coronavirus.

Medical Fact #1: *Covid-19 has a **much higher** prevalence than reported by "cases," thereby leading to a **much lower** fatality rate than reported.*

Covid-19 data will be sifted through for years to come. We don't know exactly how many people have been and are infected, although we have reason to believe that number is **vastly larger** than reported. We also don't know exactly how many people have died from

---

[18] From the AAPS (Association of American Physicians and Surgeons) May 2020 newsletter, "Virus and Resistance," Vol 76, no 5. As to the "highly contagious" comment, this has been debatable. Per the source in footnote 102, the contagion rate among household contacts of Covid-positive patients was only 3.7%!

[19] This was a phrase used by President Ronald Reagan in his 2nd Inaugural Address on January 21, 1985.

(not with) Covid, but we have reason to believe that number is **much smaller** than reported. Let me explain.

We have all gotten used to the "number of cases" reported by the media as well as various infometers and worldometers available at our fingertips.[20] These *number of cases* (the denominator in the fraction) have been consistently presented against *number of deaths* (the numerator in the fraction). For example, as of this writing, the CDC records the total US cases of 5,972,356 against the total US deaths of 182,622. Simple math shows this to be a presumed 3.1% mortality rate, which is the number of infected people who have died from Covid.[21] But is this an accurate representation of mortality?

I have a stack of positive patient Covid swab reports in a bin behind my desk. While occasionally entire households got swabbed, typically only one family member was tested, with the assumption that their result represented the entire household. We know that in many cases, the entire household contracted Covid-19, but in many cases only one family member was swabbed. That one positive result counts as one case. However, in the large families represented in our office,

---

[20] These words were not really a part of common parlance until Covid! I needed to add them to my Word dictionary.

[21] Today is 8/31/2020, as reported at https://covid.cdc.gov/covid-data-tracker/#cases. For math-challenged readers, 182,622 deaths divided by 5,972,356 = 0.0305 or 3.1%. This percentage has fluctuated. For example, *The Wall Street Journal* reported a national mortality rate of 5.5% on 4/23/20 (page A4). The WHO's numbers as of 8/30/2020 show a 3.4% mortality rate (https://www.who.int/emergencies/diseases/novel-coronavirus-2019) which is consistent with the 3.4% estimated rate published by WHO in early March 2020 (available at various sources).

the *actual* positive rate is 5 to 10 times higher than reported! That makes the denominator in our fraction *much higher*. But is that unique to our office where our patients come from large families?

Not at all! It turns out that emerging data confirms this.

- Antibody testing[22] of 3,300 patients in Santa Clara County, California found that 2.8% of the residents had positive antibodies, i.e. had already had Covid-19. This implied that 54,000 residents had been infected, which was <u>54 times</u> the predicted 1,000. Through April 22, 2020, 94 people died from Covid-19 in this County. "...94 deaths out of 54,000 infections correspond to an <u>infection fatality rate of 0.17%</u> in Santa Clara County [emphasis mine]."[23] In an opinion piece in the *Wall Street Journal*, Andrew Bogan comments, "the authors estimate that in Santa Clara County the true infection fatality rate is somewhere in the range of 0.12% to 0.2%–far closer to

---

[22] Otherwise known as seroprevalence testing, which is an antibody test, looking for the prevalence of antibodies to SARS-CoV-2 in the blood.

[23] Available online at https://www.medrxiv.org/content/10.1101/2020.04.14.20062463v2. Official citation is COVID-19 Antibody Seroprevalence in Santa Clara County, California Eran Bendavid, Bianca Mulaney, Neeraj Sood, Soleil Shah, Emilia Ling, Rebecca Bromley-Dulfano, Cara Lai, Zoe Weissberg, Rodrigo Saavedra-Walker, James Tedrow, Dona Tversky, Andrew Bogan, Thomas Kupiec, Daniel Eichner, Ribhav Gupta, John Ioannidis, Jay Bhattacharya
medRxiv 2020.04.14.20062463; doi: https://doi.org/10.1101/2020.04.14.20062463. Note this is a pre-print article which hasn't been peer-reviewed (although 17 authors contributed to this study).

seasonal influenza than to the original, case-based estimates."[24]

- Antibody testing of 16,025 people between March 23 and May 12, 2020 from 10 locations[25] across the country found positive antibodies in 1 to 6.9% of people, meaning infections were 6 to 24 times higher than reported cases. Seven of the 10 sites showed "an estimated greater than 10 times more SARS-CoV-2 infections occurred than the number of reported cases."[26]

- Dr. Robert Redfield, CDC director, stated in a conference call with reporters on June 25, 2020, "Our best estimate right now is that for every case that's reported, there actually are 10 other infections."[27] That equates to a 10 times higher actual rate of infection than reported.

- Antibody testing done on April 10 & 11, 2020 among 865 adults in Los Angeles County, California showed prevalence

---

[24] *Wall Street Journal*, April 17, 2020, available at https://www.wsj.com/articles/new-data-suggest-the-coronavirus-isnt-as-deadly-as-we-thought-11587155298?mod=searchresults&page=1&pos=4.

[25] The regions were San Francisco Bay area; Connecticut; South Florida; Louisiana; Minneapolis-St. Paul-St. Cloud metro area; Missouri; New York City metro area; Philadelphia metro area; Utah; and western Washington state.

[26] Havers FP, Reed C, Lim T, et al. Seroprevalence of Antibodies to SARS-CoV-2 in 10 Sites in the United States, March 23-May 12, 2020. *JAMA Intern Med.* Published online July 21, 2020. doi:10.1001/jamainternmed.2020.4130.

[27] https://www.nbcnews.com/health/health-news/cdc-says-covid-19-cases-u-s-may-be-10-n1232134, accessed 9/1/20. Also at https://www.washingtonpost.com/health/2020/06/25/coronavirus-cases-10-times-larger/, accessed 9/1/2020.

rates of 4.65%. This "estimate implies that approximately 367,000 adults had SARS-CoV-2 antibodies, which is sub-stantially greater [just shy of 44 times greater!] than the 8,430 cumulative number of confirmed infections in the county on April 10. Therefore, fatality rates based on confirmed cases may be higher than rates based on number of infections [em-phases and comments added]."[28]

- John P. A. Ioannidis, professor of medicine, epidemiology, and population health at Stanford, surveyed 50 population studies of at least 500 patients each which had either been peer-reviewed or were in preprint form. As of July 11, 2020, he estimated the infection fatality rate (IFR) at 0.27% (cor-rected to 0.24%).[29]

So, Dr. Fauci was right! Early on, he wrote in an editorial in *The New England Journal of Medicine (NEJM)* as early as February 28, 2020:

On the basis of a case definition requiring a diagnosis of pneumonia, the currently reported case fatality rate is ap-proximately 2%. In another article in the *Journal*, Guan et al. report mortality of 1.4% among 1099 patients with la-boratory-confirmed Covid-19; these patients had a wide

---

[28] Sood N, Simon P, Ebner P, et al. Seroprevalence of SARS-CoV-2–Specific Antibodies Among Adults in Los Angeles County, California, on April 10-11, 2020. *JAMA*. 2020;323(23):2425–2427. doi:10.1001/jama.2020.8279

[29] John Ioannidis. The infection fatality rate of COVID-19 inferred from seroprevalence data. medRxiv 2020.05.13.20101253; doi: https://doi.org/10.1101/2020.05.13.20101253

spectrum of disease severity. If one assumes that the number of asymptomatic or minimally symptomatic cases is several times as high [we now know it is *much* higher] as the number of reported cases, the case fatality rate may be considerably less than 1%. This suggests that the overall clinical consequences of Covid-19 may ultimately be more akin to those of a severe seasonal influenza (which has a case fatality rate of approximately 0.1%) or a pandemic influenza (similar to those in 1957 and 1968) rather than a disease similar to SARS or MERS, which have had case fatality rates of 9 to 10% and 36%, respectively [emphases and comments added].[30]

The dramatically higher prevalence than reported cases is used by naysayers to support containment measures and the narrative that the worst is yet to come. Afterall, if antibody testing shows only 5 to 10% of the population already had Covid-19, that means 90 to 95% did not and may yet get it! Being a "new" virus strain, perhaps that's true. But I am an optimist, and I believe this data represents great news and an exactly opposite message! Why? Because we already know how many people have died.[31] We may not know exactly how many people

---

[30] *NEJM* 2020; 382:1268-1269; March 26, 2020 print edition.

[31] Two caveats are necessary. First, every death is significant, and discussion of mortality is not meant to imply a devaluing of life. However, one must use epidemiological data to make best decisions. Second, we know that there has been much "cooking of the books" when it comes to Covid-19 death reporting. For example, an Amish patient told me of a scooter death in their community that was asked to be counted as a Covid death! We've all heard too many stories like this. It's important to distinguish between dying *from* Covid-19 versus dying *with* Covid-19.

have Covid, but we certainly know how many people have *died*. In the examples cited above, the increased prevalence ranges from 6 to 54 times greater than reported cases. Let's calculate the mortality rate using the CDC cases cited on page 67:

- 182,622 deaths/5,972,356 cases =   **3.1%**
- 182,622 deaths/59,723,560 cases (the CDC 10x) = **0.3%**
- 182,622 deaths/179,170,680 cases (30x)[32] =   **0.1%**

The average annual mortality rate of influenza in the USA over the past 9 years is 0.132%.[33] Keep in mind Dr. Fauci's comments above regarding other case fatality rates of 10 to 36%. The 1918 influenza pandemic known as the Spanish flu infected 500 million people worldwide with an estimated 20 to 50 million people dying.[34] This is a mortality rate of 4 to 10%. It should be noted that the Centre for Evidence-Based Medicine (CEBM) at the University of Oxford estimates the infection fatality rate (IFR) at 0.1 to 0.41%. They suggest an average IFR of 0.28% but clarify that "this IFR is likely an overestimate."[35] In putting all this data together, it turns out that my simple

---

[32] I am using 30x in this example because it is the median of the 6 to 54 times range.

[33] Figures are available at https://www.cdc.gov/flu/about/burden/index.html, accessed 9/1/20. There are 9 years of flu season data listed, beginning in 2010 and ending in 2019. I simply took an average of the estimate deaths divided by the estimated cases of symptomatic illness.

[34] See https://www.history.com/news/spanish-flu-second-wave-resurgence, accessed 9/1/2020.

[35] See https://www.cebm.net/covid-19/global-covid-19-case-fatality-rates/, accessed 9/1/2020.

country doctor clinical gut prediction in early April that this is akin to a bad case of the flu is actually correct![36]

The CDC releases weekly provisional death counts for COVID-19. Cumulative data from 2/1/2020 through 8/22/2020 revealed the following:[37]

Age	# of Deaths
Under 1 year	17
1 to 4 years	12
5 to 14 years	28
15 to 24 years	280
25 to 34 years	1,257
35 to 44 years	3,301
45 to 54 years	8,648
55 to 64 years	20,655
65 to 74 years	34,980
75 to 84 years	43,392
85 years +	51,710
	164,280

8.2%
232,463,605 people
(71% of population)

91.8%
94,703,829 people
(29% of population)

---

[36] One will often see a 99.8% survival rate mentioned. While "fact-checkers" will routinely debunk this statistic as inaccurate and misleading, if one subtracts the average IFR outlined above, you essentially have a 99.8% survival rate. So yes, I would argue that 99.8% *is* accurate. A look beneath the surface of "fact-checkers" will reveal that most all are controlled by Big Tech, and Big Tech has a vested interest in the information that you are privy to. But that's another book!

[37] At https://www.cdc.gov/nchs/nvss/vsrr/covid_weekly/index.htm?fbclid=IwAR3R6Q-XItp-t1LFhMznW746ADK-Cz8CPXqSOztEQhA1vXKIISwcr9PobcI, accessed 9/1/2020.

These numbers show what we would expect: as you get older, the risk of dying from Covid-19 dramatically increases. Given the fact that Covid-19 is a respiratory disease, this is not surprising, as pneumonia broadly has been categorized as the "old man's friend."[38]

In the above CDC report under "Comorbidities" and Table 3, there was a fascinating statement: "<u>For 6% of the deaths, COVID-19 was the only cause mentioned</u>. For deaths with conditions or causes in addition to COVID-19, on average, there were 2.6 additional conditions or causes per death [emphasis added]." Much has been made of this 6%. In all fairness to the data, this simply means that only 6% of the death certificates listed Covid-19 as the only cause of death. When physicians fill out death certificates, they usually always list contributing causes of death. In the 6%, there were no other causes listed, either because there were none or they hadn't been documented. The other 94% had listed contributing causes. While this doesn't necessarily mean that only 6% of the deaths were from Covid-19, it *certainly* shows that significant comorbidities contributed (and likely were causative) to death, and that many of these patients were likely dying *with* and not *from* Covid.

---

[38] This has broadly been attributed to Sir William Osler, the father of modern medicine, who himself died at age 70 of pneumonia. He wrote in his 1892 *The Principles and Practice of Medicine*, "In children and in healthy adults the outlook is good. In the debilitated, in drunkards and in the aged the chances are against recovery. So fatal is it in the latter class [i.e. the elderly] that it has been termed the natural end of the old man." From https://pneumonia.biomedcentral.com/articles/10.1186/s41479-018-0052-7, accessed 9/1/2020.

Medical Fact #2: *There are numerous comorbidities associated with Covid-19 whose severity increases with age, making Covid-19 a relatively benign disease for most people.*

A "comorbidity" is a medical term for a disease existing alongside another one. The above CDC data clearly shows this: there was an average of 2.6 additional diseases beside Covid-19 on death certificates. The table on the previous page also shows this, as one is likely to have more health problems (i.e. comorbidities) as one ages. You can see that the vast majority—nearly 92%—of deaths occurred in patients over age 55. *Yet nearly three-quarters of the country who were at very low risk overall were locked down.* When you look back at the table, it certainly makes one ask the question why the onerous back to school and college restrictions remain in effect.

Since New York was one of the epicenters of the pandemic, data from there is revealing. A study of 5,700 patients between March 1 and April 4, 2020 with an average age of 63 hospitalized in New York City with Covid-19 showed the most common comorbidities were hypertension (56.6%), obesity (41.7%), and diabetes (33.8%).[39] According to Table 1, only 350 (6.1%) of these had no comorbidities and 4,991 (88%) had more than one.[40] "As of midnight on April 6, there had been 5,489 fatalities caused by COVID-19 in the state, of

---

[39] Richardson S, Hirsch JS, Narasimhan M, et al. Presenting Characteristics, Comorbidities, and Outcomes Among 5700 Patients Hospitalized With COVID-19 in the New York City Area. *JAMA.* 2020;323(20):2052–2059. doi:10.1001/jama.2020.6775.
[40] It's *very interesting* that this 6% from New York City is identical to the 6% noted in the above CDC report who had Covid-19 only.

which 86.2% (4,732) had at least one underlying condition, the New York State Department of Health reported April 7."[41] Per the online *Chest Physician*™, the 10 most common comorbidities in Covid-19 fatalities were diabetes (37.3%), hyperlipidemia (18.5%), coronary artery disease (12.4%), renal disease (11%), dementia (9.1%), COPD (8.3%), cancer (8.1%), atrial fibrillation (7.1%), and heart failure (7.1%).[42] This site also notes that 63% of all Covid-related deaths involved patients age 70 years or older.

In a correspondence piece in *The Lancet*, the authors writing from Peking University People's Hospital in Beijing warned:

> More attention should be paid to comorbidities in the treatment of COVID-19. In the literature, COVID-19 is characterised [sic] by the symptoms of viral pneumonia such as fever, fatigue, dry cough, and lymphopenia. Many of the older patients who become severely ill have evidence of underlying illnesses such as cardiovascular disease, liver disease, kidney disease, or malignant tumours. These patients often die of their original comorbidities; we therefore need to accurately evaluate all original comorbidities of individuals with COVID-19 [emphasis added].[43]

---

[41] At https://www.mdedge.com/chestphysician/article/220457/coronavirus-updates/comorbidities-rule-new-yorks-covid-19-deaths, accessed 9/2/2020.

[42] Ibid.

[43] Comorbidities and multi-organ injuries in the treatment of COVID-19. Tianbing Wang et al. *The Lancet* Vol 395 Iss 10228, E52, March 21, 2020; https://doi.org/10.1016/S0140-6736(20)30558-4. For readers not familiar with *The Lancet*, it is one of the world's premier and most-respected British medical journals.

An online CME[44] activity notes, "Although COVID-19 appears to be highly transmissible, only a small percentage of people seems to develop severe illness, and an even smaller number die from the infection. However, statistics to date suggest worse prognosis with COVID-19 infection among people with diabetes and cardiovascular disease (CVD) [emphasis added]."[45] The CME activity goes on to cite a JAMA[46] study of 44,672 positive Covid-19 Chinese patients in which *81% were mild cases* (defined as no pneumonia or mild pneumonia), 14% were severe (with significant shortness of breath and decreased oxygen levels of 93% or lower), and 5% were critical (with respiratory failure and/or multi-organ failure). Of the 1,023 deaths which occurred, nearly half (49%) were in the critical category, 14.8% were age 80 years or older, and 8% were age 70 to 79. As with other studies, preexisting comorbidities such as CVD (10.5%), diabetes (7.3%), chronic respiratory disease (6.3%), hypertension (6%), and cancer (5.6%) significantly contributed to an elevated death rate. The activity further notes "that diabetes is associated with double or triple the risk

---

[44] CME is continuing medical education, required for physicians to maintain their license.

[45] Are diabetes, CVD associated with worse COVID-19 prognosis? Barclay & Nyarko, released 3/4/2020, available at https://www.medscape.org/viewarticle/926097, accessed 9/1/2020.

[46] *Journal of the American Medical Association*, established in 1883. The journal reference isWu Z, McGoogan JM. Characteristics of and Important Lessons From the Coronavirus Disease 2019 (COVID-19) Outbreak in China: Summary of a Report of 72 314 Cases From the Chinese Center for Disease Control and Prevention. *JAMA*. 2020;323(13):1239–1242. doi:10.1001/jama.2020.2648.

for infection from COVID-19, independent of CVD or other medical comorbidities."[47]

Note the underlined sentence on the previous page. When any of our patients had a positive Covid swab, the lab sent us a copy of the positive results along with a notification to patients, which included this message:

> Most patients with COVID-19 **DO NOT** require specific medical attention or hospitalization and can manage their symptoms at home.[48]

A study of 1,590 patients hospitalized across mainline China with Covid-19 between December 11, 2019 and January 31, 2020 showed hypertension (16.9%) and diabetes (8.2%) to be the most common comorbidities.[49] A study from Mexico showed that obesity was the strongest comorbidity.[50]

---

[47] Ibid.

[48] This was from one of our local hospitals, is entirely correct, and a message which has been *dramatically understated* or simply *un*stated.

[49] Comorbidity and its impact on 1590 patients with Covid-19 in China: A Nationwide Analysis. Wei-jie Guan et al (47 authors); *European Respiratory Journal* Jan 2020, 2000547; **DOI:** 10.1183/13993003.00547-2020.

[50] Obesity is the comorbidity more strongly associated for Covid-19 in Mexico. A case-control study. Eduardo Hernández-Garduño. *Obesity Research & Clinical Practice*, Vol 14 Issue 4 (Jul-Aug 2020) 375-379; https://doi.org/10.1016/j.orcp.2020.06.001.

Medical Fact #3: *Coronavirus is not new.*

The first human coronavirus was identified in 1965.[51] It belongs to the family Coronaviridae and measures approximately 120 nanometers (nm) or 0.12 microns (μm). *Please note this size, as it is critical to what follows.* It is so-named because of the glycoprotein club-shaped spikes attached to the virus' outer envelope, giving it a "crown-like" or *coronal* appearance. We've all become quite familiar with this picture over the past number of months. Some coronaviruses affect animals, such as cats, camels, and cattle. Some affect humans. A particularly virulent strain known as SARS (sudden acute respiratory syndrome) was identified in China in 2002 and by 2003 had spread to 8,098 people in 28 countries causing 774 deaths.[52] As noted by Dr. Fauci above (see footnote #30), it had a case fatality rate of about 10%. Another similar coronavirus known as MERS (Middle Eastern Respiratory Syndrome) began in Saudi Arabia in 2012. It affected approximately 2,500 people causing 858 deaths. It was less contagious but more deadly with a case fatality rate of 36%. When SARS-CoV-2 was identified (see footnote #1), it was originally called "novel" coronavirus because it was a new strain. This was, in my opinion, a poor name because it implied to the general public an entirely new virus strain. This is the *most contagious* coronavirus to date, but by far the *least*

---

[51] See https://www.webmd.com/lung/coronavirus-history, accessed 9/2/2020.
[52] See https://www.cdc.gov/sars/about/fs-sars.html, accessed 9/2/2020.

deadly, as evidenced by the data presented above. Indeed, as WebMD states, "most coronaviruses aren't dangerous."[53]

We now transition to some of the myths being perpetrated[54] on the general public.

Myth #1: *Masks are effective.*

I will show my hand right from the outset—I am opposed to universal mask-wearing, *because there is no credible medical evidence to support it.*[55] I know that supporters of masked mandates will immediately push back and ask if I haven't read "such and such a study" which shows that "mask use can reduce transmission by 30% or more"[56] or that universal mask-wearing by all members of the population would stamp out coronavirus in a few short weeks? Have I not read the *JAMA* report that "universal masking at MGB [Mass General Brigham] was

---

[53] See https://www.webmd.com/lung/coronavirus, accessed 9/2/2020.

[54] I use this word intentionally.

[55] I take full responsibility for this statement and am willing to place my professional reputation on the line in support of this statement. I am not necessarily recommending that health care workers not wear masks during exposure. However, LuAnne and I have never worn masks in our office during seasonal sickness and we have <u>not</u> worn masks during Covid, apart from a brief 2-week period early on.

[56] From https://covid19.healthdata.org/united-states-of-america?view=total-deaths&tab=trend, accessed ~8/29/20. This is from the widely criticized IHME (Institute for Health Metrics and Evaluation) at the University of Washington. It should be noted that in early 2017, IHME received a pledge of $279 million from the Bill & Melinda Gates Foundation, according to https://www.gatesfoundation.org/Media-Center/Press-Releases/2017/01/IHME-Announcement, accessed 9/3/20. It should also be noted that the above quotation has no solid scientific documentation. Data sources to support this statement are behavioral and social media/science <u>surveys</u>, not actual data.

associated with a significantly lower rate of SARS-CoV-2 positivity among HCWs [health care workers]"?[57]

The answer is both *yes* and *no*! *Yes*, I'm familiar with these reports and I'm reading the hard copy of the one as I write. But *no*, in the sense that all of this flies in the face of what we knew to be true prior to March 2020. Many of the "new" studies showing efficacy of masks are not studies at all but rather computer-generated mathematical predictor models showing what *could* be true but not what *is* true. Just as I smelled a rat in early April, I smell a rat in all of this. As C. S. Lewis wrote in deadpan sarcasm, "There has been a revolution of opinion on that in educated circles"![58] He also wrote, "I cannot love a lie. I cannot love the thing which is not."[59] Let me explain.

The Lancet published "Rational use of face masks in the COVID-19 pandemic" online on March 20, 2020 and in the May

---

[57] Wang X, Ferro EG, Zhou G, Hashimoto D, Bhatt DL. Association Between Universal Masking in a Health Care System and SARS-CoV-2 Positivity Among Health Care Workers. *JAMA*. 2020;324(7):703–704. doi:10.1001/jama.2020.12897. (This is actually from the *JAMA* hard copy in my office, journal dated 8/18/2020!)

[58] Lewis, C.S. (1946, 1974, 1996). *The Great Divorce*. New York: Simon & Schuster, A Touchstone Book., p. 25. While I'm all for learning new things and keeping an open mind, I've been in my profession long enough to distrust recommendations that are polar opposites from previous ones. *Evidence-based medicine* (EBM) supposedly looks at evidence and makes recommendations. Here's a simple example. For years, newborn moms were told to use alcohol on the umbilical stumps of their newborns. Now, that is *not* recommended because of new evidence. And I ask, was any harm done to any of the babies whose mothers did that for years?! Not to my knowledge.

[59] Ibid, p. 116.

2020 print edition.[60] Here were the recommendations from various countries on the use of masks as documented individually from their various departments of health:

- WHO: "If you are healthy, you only need to wear a mask if you are taking care of a person with suspected SARS-CoV-2 infection."
- Singapore: "Wear a mask if you have respiratory symptoms, such as a cough or runny nose."
- Japan: "The effectiveness of wearing a face mask to protect yourself from contracting viruses is thought to be limited."
- USA: "Centers for Disease Control and Prevention does not recommend that people who are well wear a face mask (including respirators) to protect themselves from respiratory diseases, including COVID-19."
- USA: "US Surgeon General urged people on Twitter to stop buying face masks."
- UK: "Face masks play a very important role in places such as hospitals, but there is very little evidence of widespread benefit for members of the public."
- Germany: "There is not enough evidence to prove that wearing a surgical mask significantly reduces a healthy person's risk of becoming infected while wearing it. According to WHO,

---

[60] Feng et al. "Rational use of face masks in the COVID-19 pandemic," *The Lancet Respiratory Medicine*, online March 20, 2020; Volume 8, Issue 5, P434-436, May 01, 2020. https://doi.org/10.1016/S2213-2600(20)30134-X.

wearing a mask in situations where it is not recommended to do so can create a false sense of security because it might lead to neglecting fundamental hygiene measures, such as proper hand hygiene."[61]

As recent as March 4, 2020, recommendations on a *JAMA* patient page stated: "Face makes should not be worn by healthy individuals to protect themselves from acquiring respiratory infection because *there is no evidence that face masks worn by healthy individuals are effective in preventing people from becoming ill* [emphasis mine]."[62] In an interview on 60 Minutes on March 8, 2020, Dr. Fauci stated, "Right now in the United States, people should not be walking around with masks…There's no reason to be walking around with a mask. When you're in the middle of an outbreak wearing a mask might make people feel a little bit better, and it might even block a droplet, but it's not providing the perfect protection that people think that it is. And often, there are unintended consequences; people keep fiddling with the mask and they keep touching their face…"[63]

These recommendations are very clear and quite difficult to interpret any other way: *masks are not recommended for healthy people.*

---

[61] Only China and Hong Kong had various recommendations for mask wearing based on risk of infection or being in public. Even China stated that "people of very low risk of infection do not have to wear a mask or can wear non-medical mask (such as cloth mask)."

[62] Desai & Mehrotra, "Medical Masks," *JAMA*. 2020;323(15):1517-1518. doi:10.1001/jama.2020.2331, published March 4, 2020.

[63] My own transcript from YouTube, available at https://www.youtube.com/watch?v=PRa6t_e7dgI, accessed 9/12/2020.

In addition, the protective benefit of facemasks even in medical settings has been disputed in the medical literature for some time.

Tom Jefferson is an epidemiologist and honorary research fellow at University of Oxford's Centre for Evidence-Based Medicine (CEBM), which is directed by professor of evidence-based medicine Carl Heneghan. They recently revised some of their original work (from 2007) on how effective barriers are to transmitting infections. They note, "Evidence from 14 trials on the use of masks vs. no masks was disappointing: it showed no effect in either healthcare workers or in community settings. We could also find no evidence of a difference between the N95 and other types of masks..."[64, 65] In all fairness to them, they state that "our findings cannot be the final word." They also state that "there is no evidence of effectiveness" of cloth masks. In the same article, Jefferson and Heneghan cite an 84 literature reference review concluding in the first line of the abstract, "The use of

---

[64] Jefferson & Heneghan, "COVID-19—Masks on or off?" April 17, 2020, on CEBM website (https://www.cebm.net/covid-19/covid-19-masks-on-or-off/), originally accessed around 4/25/2020, re-accessed 9/5/2020.

[65] Physical interventions to interrupt or reduce the spread of respiratory viruses. Part 1 - Face masks, eye protection and person distancing: systematic review and meta-analysis Tom Jefferson, Mark Jones, Lubna A Al Ansari, Ghada Bawazeer, Elaine Beller, Justin Clark, John Conly, Chris Del Mar, Elisabeth Dooley, Eliana Ferroni, Paul Glasziou, Tammy Hoffman, Sarah Thorning, Mieke Van Driel medRxiv 2020.03.30.20047217; doi: https://doi.org/10.1101/2020.03.30.20047217. In the abstract, the authors state: "Compared to no masks there was no reduction of influenza-like (ILI) cases or influenza for masks in the general population, nor in healthcare workers. There was no difference between surgical masks and N95 respirators [for ILI or influenza]...All trials were conducted during seasonal ILI activity."

protective facemasks (PFMs) <u>negatively impacts respiratory and dermal mechanisms</u> of human thermoregulation through impairment of convection, evaporation, and radiation processes [emphasis added]."[66]

The first randomized controlled trial of cloth masks (among healthcare workers) was published in 2015. It compared cloth masks, medical masks, and a control group (unspecified mask wearing). It showed that "the rates of all infection outcomes were highest in the cloth mask arm, with the rate of ILI [influenza-like illness] statistically significantly higher in the cloth mask arm compared with the medical mask arm [and the control arm]...<u>Penetration of cloth mask by particles was almost 97%</u> and medical masks 44% [emphasis added]." The authors concluded that "the results caution against the use of cloth masks....Moisture retention, reuse of cloth masks and poor filtration may result in increased risk of infection."[67]

In a very small study of 4 patients published April 6, 2020 in the *Annals of Internal Medicine*, the authors concluded:

---

[66] Raymond J. Roberge, Jung-Hyun Kim, Aitor Coca, Protective Facemask Impact on Human Thermoregulation: An Overview, *The Annals of Occupational Hygiene*, Volume 56, Issue 1, January 2012, Pages 102–112, https://doi.org/10.1093/annhyg/mer069.

[67] MacIntyre CR, Seale H, Dung TC, *et al* A cluster randomised trial of cloth masks compared with medical masks in healthcare workers. *BMJ Open* 2015;5:e006577. doi: 10.1136/bmjopen-2014-006577. Note that the authors to this original article provided an updated statement on 30 March 2020 (in light of Covid and shortage of PPE [personal protective equipment]) but did <u>not</u> retract any of their original observations. (Updated statement available at original citation.)

Neither surgical nor cotton masks effectively filtered SARS-CoV-2 during coughs by infected patients...Oberg and Brousseau demonstrated that surgical makes did not exhibit adequate filter performance against aerosols measuring 0.9, 2.0, and 3.1 μm in diameter. Lee and colleagues demonstrated that particles 0.04 to 0.2 μm can penetrate surgical masks. The size of the SARS-CoV particle from the 2002-2004 outbreak was estimated as 0.08 to 0.14 μm; assuming that SARS-CoV-2 has a similar size, surgical masks are unlikely to effectively filter this virus.

Of note, we found greater contamination on the outer than the inner mask surfaces...

In conclusion, <u>both surgical and cotton masks seem to be ineffective in preventing the dissemination of SARS-CoV-2 from the coughs of patients with COVID-19</u> to the environment and external mask surface [emphasis added].[68]

---

[68] Bae, S., Kim, M. C., Kim, J. Y., Cha, H. H., Lim, J. S., Jung, J., Kim, M. J., Oh, D. K., Lee, M. K., Choi, S. H., Sung, M., Hong, S. B., Chung, J. W., & Kim, S. H. (2020). Effectiveness of Surgical and Cotton Masks in Blocking SARS-CoV-2: A Controlled Comparison in 4 Patients. *Annals of internal medicine, 173*(1), W22–W23. https://doi.org/10.7326/M20-1342 (Retraction published Ann Intern Med. 2020 Jun 2). Note the "retraction" comment! A "limit of detection" methodological weakness highlighted by readers led the editors of the *Annals* to request retraction. The authors state on the retraction site, "<u>We proposed</u> correcting the reported data with new experimental data from additional patients, <u>but the editors requested retraction</u> [emphasis added]." Any thinking person should smell a rat! Doesn't science advance itself by ongoing investigation? Would not the correct way forward have been what the authors propose—get more data, tighten up the methodological weakness, and re-publish results? The fact that the editors requested retraction rather than further investigation is **<u>highly suspicious</u>** for "let's just keep

Writing in the *Singapore Medical Journal* in 2014, Viroj Wiwanitkit writes, "Since the coronavirus is an extremely small virus, it can pass through the pores of both the surgical mask and N95 respirator."[69, 70] Note again the dimensions in the preceding quote in light of the following observations:

- SARS-CoV-2 is a virus measuring approximately 0.12μm (120 nm) in diameter.[71] Others estimate its diameter at <u>0.10 μm</u> (100 nm).[72]

---

the scientific community hoodwinked because this is heading in a direction not supported by the top-down narrative." This is an all-too-common theme: credible voices whose conclusions counter the mainstream narrative are forcibly silenced. **Neither science nor a free society will flourish in such an environment.**

[69] Wiwanitkit V. (2014). MERS-CoV, surgical mask and N95 respirators. *Singapore medical journal*, 55(9), 507. https://doi.org/10.11622/smedj.2014124.

[70] The authors of the original study reply to his comment with, "Based on the pore sizes of the protective apparatus and the size of the virus, we agree that there is probably no difference between surgical masks and N95 respirators." Chung, J. S., Ling, M. L., Seto, W. H., Ang, B. S., & Tambyah, P. A. (2014). Authors' Reply. MERS-CoV, surgical mask and N95 respirators. *Singapore medical journal*, 55(9), 507. https://doi.org/10.11622/smedj.2014125. Available on the CDC website at https://wwwnc.cdc.gov/eid/article/26/5/19-0994_article, accessed 6/14/2020, re-accessed 9/5/2020.

[71] Per https://www.pptaglobal.org/media-and-information/ppta-statements/1055-2019-novel-coronavirus-2019-ncov-and-plasma-protein-therapies, accessed 8/16/2020, re-accessed 9/5/2020.

[72] Bar-On, Y. M., Flamholz, A., Phillips, R., & Milo, R. (2020). SARS-CoV-2 (COVID-19) by the numbers. *eLife*, 9, e57309. https://doi.org/10.7554/eLife.57309.

- The "gold standard" in masks is the N95 surgical respirator. "CDC guidelines state that 3M™ Surgical N95 Respirators can be used for *M. tuberculosis* exposure control."[73] This means that the surgical N95 is approved by the CDC for stopping only <u>one</u> organism—TB (*Mycobacterium tuberculosis*). The surgical N95 also differs from the contractor's N95; the latter has an exhale valve, may or may not be fitted properly, and likely doesn't have the tight seal against the skin.

- "Mycobacterial shape within alveolar macrophages varied from shorter oval, approximately 0.5 to 1 µm in length, to the classical rods with a mean length in 2-4 µm, and long filamentous forms over 6-7 µm in length, while *Mtb* width did not change significantly."[74] In general, "the rods are <u>2-5 micrometers [µm] in length</u> and <u>0.2-0.5 µm in width</u>."[75]

- Reviewing the underlined facts above, this means that SARS-CoV-2 is ***2 to 5 times smaller*** than the approved filtering capability of a surgical N95. This is based on the <u>width</u> of the TB bacterium in comparison to the circular nature of the SARS-

[73] Per the 3M™ website at https://multimedia.3m.com/mws/media/901539O/3m-healthcare-respirators.pdf, accessed 8/16/2020, re-accessed 9/5/2020.

[74] Mycobacterium tuberculosis shape and size variations in alveolar macrophages of tuberculosis patients
Elena Ufimtseva, Natalya Eremeeva, Diana Vakhrusheva, Sergey Skornyakov. *European Respiratory Journal* Sep 2019, 54 (suppl 63) PA4605; **DOI:** 10.1183/13993003.congress-2019.PA4605.

[75] Per Kenneth Todar, PhD, *Online Textbook of Bacteriology*, available at http://textbookof-bacteriology.net/tuberculosis.html, accessed 9/5/2020.

CoV-2 molecule. (Based on the length of TB, it is 40 to 70 times larger than SARS-CoV-2!) As some of my patients have told me, it's like expecting a chain-link fence (N95) to stop a mosquito (SARS-CoV-2)!

Note these comments regarding face masks from May 2020 *Emerging Infectious Diseases* and available on the CDC website:

> In our systematic review, we identified 10 RCTs [randomized control trials] that reported estimates of the effectiveness of face masks in reducing laboratory-confirmed influenza virus infections in the community...we found no significant reduction in influenza transmission with the use of face masks. One study evaluated the use of face masks among pilgrims from Australia during the Hajj pilgrimage and reported no major difference in the risk for laboratory-confirmed influenza virus infection in the control or mask group. Two studies in university settings assessed the effectiveness of face masks for primary protection by monitoring the incidence of laboratory-confirmed influenza among student hall residents for 5 months. The overall reduction in ILI or laboratory-confirmed influenza cases in the face mask group was not significant in either studies...None of the household studies reported a significant reduction in secondary laboratory-confirmed influenza virus infections in the face mask group...[76]

---

[76] Xiao, J., Shiu, E., Gao, H., Wong, J. Y., Fong, M. W., Ryu, S....Cowling, B. J. (2020). Nonpharmaceutical Measures for Pandemic Influenza in Nonhealthcare Settings—Personal

Because our reference point to date for studying respiratory illnesses has been influenza, many of the following citations are largely regarding influenza and other URIs (upper respiratory infections).[77]

In 2009, thirty-two health care workers outside surgical suites in Asia were randomized into a group wearing masks and one not wearing masks. "Face mask use in health care workers has not been demonstrated to provide benefit in terms of cold symptoms or getting colds."[78]

A 2010 systematic literature review of 6 healthcare settings and 4 outpatient settings showed "no significant difference" in transmission of influenza between masks versus control groups in eight out of the ten studies.[79]

Protective and Environmental Measures. *Emerging Infectious Diseases, 26*(5), 967-975. https://dx.doi.org/10.3201/eid2605.190994.

[77] I am indebted to a review of the scientific literature by Denis G. Rancourt, PhD, a retired and former tenured full professor of physics (highest rank) at the University of Ottawa and now researcher for Ontario Civil Liberties Association, as cited in Rancourt D J, Masks don't work: A review of science relevant to COVID-19 policy, Technical Report, April 2020, DOI: 10.13140/RG.2.2.14320.40967/1. I did trace each of his citations to their primary sources as noted in the following footnotes. Note that all these studies were among health care workers.

[78] Jacobs JL, Ohde S, Takahashi O, Tokuda Y, Omata F, Fukui T. Use of surgical face masks to reduce the incidence of the common cold among health care workers in Japan: a randomized controlled trial. *Am J Infect Control.* 2009;37(5):417-419. doi:10.1016/j.ajic.2008.11.002.

[79] Cowling, B., Zhou, Y., Ip, D., Leung, G., & Aiello, A. (2010). Face masks to prevent transmission of influenza virus: A systematic review. *Epidemiology and Infection, 138*(4), 449-456. doi:10.1017/S0950268809991658. This data is nicely summarized in Tables 1 &

A 2011 review of "17 eligible studies" found that "none of the studies established a conclusive relationship between mask/respirator use and protection against influenza infection."[80]

A 2013 literature review showed that the use of surgical masks in the operating room had no effect on prevention of surgical site infections (SSI). Some of the literature suggested that surgical face masks increased the likelihood of infection, while "all other trials included in the systematic reviews did not demonstrate any statistically significant differences in SSI frequency between the masked and unmasked group."[81] While this is not directly applicable to Covid-19, it *does* show that masks often fail to do what we expect them to do.

The *Canadian Medical Association Journal (CMAJ)* published a review of relevant studies between January 1990 and December 2014. In reviewing 6 clinical studies and 23 surrogate exposure studies, "we found no significant difference between N95 respirators and surgical masks in associated risk of (a) laboratory-confirmed respiratory

---

2. Of the other two (out of ten studies), one showed "suboptimal use of standard precautions during high-risk procedures [was] associated with higher risk of infection" and the other was a 1918 Boston open-air hospital with a "low case-fatality rate [which] could be associated with use of natural ventilation and gauze face masks."

[80] bin-Reza et al. (2012) The use of masks and respirators to prevent transmission of influenza: a systematic review of the scientific evidence. *Influenza and Other Respiratory Viruses* 6(4), 257–267. DOI:10.1111/j.1750-2659.2011.00307.x, www.influenzajournal.com.

[81] Use of Surgical Masks in the Operating Room: A Review of the Clinical Effectiveness and Guidelines [Internet]. Ottawa (ON): Canadian Agency for Drugs and Technologies in Health; 2013 Nov 19. SUMMARY OF EVIDENCE. Available from: https://www.ncbi.nlm.nih.gov/books/NBK195776/.

infection; (b) influenza-like illness; or (c) reported workplace absenteeism."[82]

A 2017 review of 6 RCTs and 23 observational studies (after starting with 2,333 articles) yielded the following: "Our analysis confirms the effectiveness of medical masks and respirators against SARS. Disposable, cotton, or paper masks are not recommended [emphasis added]....Overall, the evidence of inform policies on mask use in HCWs is poor, with a small number of studies that is prone to reporting biases [i.e. dependent on self-reporting]."[83]

In 2019, randomized clinical control trial of 2,862 health care personnel concluded: "...N95 respirators vs medical masks as worn by participants in this trial resulted in no significant difference in the incidence of laboratory-confirmed influenza."[84]

Early this year, six RCTs representing 9,171 participants concluded that "there were no statistically significant differences in preventing laboratory-confirmed influenza, laboratory-confirmed

---

[82] Effectiveness of N95 respirators versus surgical masks in protecting health care workers from acute respiratory infection: a systematic review and meta-analysis. Jeffrey D. Smith, Colin C. MacDougall, Jennie Johnstone, Ray A. Copes, Brian Schwartz, Gary E. Garber. *CMAJ* May 2016, 188 (8) 567-574; **DOI:** 10.1503/cmaj.150835

[83] Vittoria Offeddu, Chee Fu Yung, Mabel Sheau Fong Low, Clarence C Tam, Effectiveness of Masks and Respirators Against Respiratory Infections in Healthcare Workers: A Systematic Review and Meta-Analysis, *Clinical Infectious Diseases*, Volume 65, Issue 11, 1 December 2017, Pages 1934–1942, https://doi.org/10.1093/cid/cix681.

[84] Radonovich LJ, Simberkoff MS, Bessesen MT, et al. N95 Respirators vs Medical Masks for Preventing Influenza Among Health Care Personnel: A Randomized Clinical Trial. *JAMA*. 2019;322(9):824–833. doi:10.1001/jama.2019.11645.

respiratory viral infections, laboratory-confirmed respiratory infection and influenza like illness using N95 respirators and surgical masks....The use of N95 respirators compared with surgical masks is not associated with a lower risk of laboratory-confirmed influenza...[and] suggests that N95 respirators should not be recommended for [the] general public..."[85]

So why the shift? Why did the WHO, the CDC, and departments of health suddenly—almost overnight and almost universally—start recommending that healthy people start wearing masks? Why did previous websites recommending *against* mask-wearing get replaced by sites *promoting* mask-wearing? Why did the Surgeon General switch from telling the public to stop buying masks[86] to showing on video how to make a homemade mask out of an old scarf?[87] Why did the purpose of a mask to "protect me" (i.e. *I* wear a mask to protect *me* from germs) shift to the purpose of a mask to "protect you" (i.e. *I* wear a mask to prevent *you* from getting sick)? If "there is no evidence" that a face mask prevents a well person from becoming ill, how can there now be evidence in a few short weeks that a face mask prevents a well person from making another well person ill?! It begs the question what in our medical understanding changed so dramatically in such a short time to promote an entirely opposite recommendation? I

---

[85] Long Y, Hu T, Liu L, et al. Effective-ness of N95 respirators versus surgical masks against influenza: A systematic review and meta-analysis. *J Evid Based Med.*2020;13:93–101. https://doi.org/10.1111/jebm.12381.

[86] Review footnote #60.

[87] This is available widely across the internet.

submit to you that *nothing* changed in our scientific understanding. Which leads us to the second myth.

Myth #2: *We are all asymptomatic spreaders of Covid and therefore must "socially distance" ourselves from others.*

It would be reasonable to assume that public health experts were aware of the essential ineffectiveness of face masks based on the above data. It is also fair to say that the term "social distancing" was probably unheard of by most people prior to 2020. I certainly had never heard of it. Now, unfortunately, it has become common parlance.

Unless you are a statistician, you probably also had not heard the term "flattening the curve." But then, we all heard of the initial predictions from Imperial College London and the IHME (Institute for Health Metrics and Evaluation) from the University of Washington. These mathematical and epidemiological models have been widely debated and criticized. Threats of quarantine led to the world's first toilet paper shortage, and suggestions that SARS-CoV-2 could possibly live on hard surfaces for hours to days as well as be transmitted by airborne droplets for up to 6 (some suggested 27[88]) feet led to the sanitizer shortage. And then, almost with the force of a moral imperative, all were expected to "lock down" at home, socially distance

---

[88] Bourouiba L. Turbulent Gas Clouds and Respiratory Pathogen Emissions: Potential Implications for Reducing Transmission of COVID-19. *JAMA.* 2020;323(18):1837–1838. doi:10.1001/jama.2020.4756.

from friends and family, wear masks, "stay safe," and "do our part" because "we're all in this together" in an effort to flatten the curve.[89]

Quarantine is not a new public health strategy. It was certainly practiced in biblical times for lepers.[90] "Organized institutional responses to disease control began during the plague epidemic of 1347-1352"[91] in Europe, according to Eugenia Tognotti, a biomedical researcher at the University of Sassari in Italy. She further writes:

> Quarantine…strategies have always been much debated, perceived as intrusive, and accompanied in every age and under all political regimes by an undercurrent of suspicion, distrust, and riots. These strategic measures have raised (and continue to raise) a variety of political, economic, social, and ethical issues. In the face of dramatic health crisis, individual rights have often been trampled in the name of public good. The use of segregation or isolation to separate persons *suspected of being infected* [emphasis mine] has frequently violated the liberty of outwardly healthy persons…"

---

[89] It's important to note that "flattening the curve" was originally designed *to prevent hospitals from being overrun* by keeping the public from circulating so that illness would not spread. While hard-hit areas certainly had overflowing ICUs, many hospitals across the country never experienced the expected inundation. That is certainly the case in 5 large hospital systems in my immediate practice area.

[90] It wasn't until the twentieth century that leprosy was discovered to not be a contagious disease, thanks to the heroic work of Dr. Paul Brand and others.

[91] Tognotti E. (2013). Lessons from the history of quarantine, from plague to influenza A. *Emerging infectious diseases, 19*(2), 254–259. https://doi.org/10.3201/eid1902.120312.

And that is the key—"suspected of being infected." And therein lies the rub, because both national masking and social distancing strategies are predicated on the unfounded assumption that we are all suspected of being infected. That is certainly how it's portrayed by the media. So why do I say it's unfounded and even further untrue?

Some of the first returning travelers from Wuhan, China were thought to be asymptomatic transmitters of Covid-19. Bill Gates wrote a perspective piece in the *NEJM* in late February 2020 stating, "There is also strong evidence that it can be transmitted by people who are just mildly ill or even presymptomatic."[92] His reference was a correspondence piece signed by 20 physician-scientists and published online by *NEJM* on February 18 and later in the print edition of March 26, 2020. Their language was far less certain:

> ...epidemiologic *uncertainty* regarding *possible* transmission of the virus by asymptomatically or subclinically symptomatic infected persons. It is *unclear* whether persons who show no signs or symptoms of respiratory infection shed SARS-CoV-2.

---

[92] Gates B. Responding to Covid-19—A Once-in-a-Century Pandemic? *N Engl J Med* 2020; 382:1677-1679, April 30, 2020 (online Feb 28, 2020). DOI: 10.1056/NEJMp2003762. It is curious to me that Gates is considered a medical expert and given space in one of the world's premier medical journals.

We discovered that shedding of potentially infectious virus *may* occur in persons who have no fever and no signs or only minor signs of infection [all emphases mine].[93]

The March 12, 2020 edition of *Eurosurveillance* states:

Currently, *there is no clear evidence that COVID-19 asymptomatic persons can transmit SARS-CoV-2*, but there is accumulating evidence indicating that a substantial fraction of SARS-CoV-2 infected individuals are asymptomatic." They further state "that transmission of SARS-CoV-2 by asymptomatic or paucisymptomatic cases *may* be possible, even though *there is no clear evidence as yet* of asymptomatic transmission [emphases mine].[94]

The April 10, 2020 edition of the CDC's *MMWR* notes:

...the existence of presymptomatic or asymptomatic transmission would present difficult challenges to contact tracing. Such transmission modes *have not been definitely documented for COVID-19*, although cases of presymptomatic and asymptomatic transmissions *have been reported* in China

[93] Hoehl et al. Evidence of SARS-CoV-2 Infection in Returning Travelers from Wuhan, China, *N Engl J Med* 2020; 382:1278-1280, March 26, 2020 (online Feb 18, 2020). DOI: 10.1056/NEJMc200189.

[94] Mizumoto, K., Kagaya, K., Zarebski, A., & Chowell, G. (2020). Estimating the asymptomatic proportion of coronavirus disease 2019 (COVID-19) cases on board the Diamond Princess cruise ship, Yokohama, Japan, 2020. *Euro surveillance : bulletin Europeen sur les maladies transmissibles = European communicable disease bulletin*, 25(10), 2000180. https://doi.org/10.2807/1560-7917.ES.2020.25.10.2000180. (This journal is "Europe's journal on infectious disease epidemiology, prevention and control since 1996.")

and *possibly occurred* in a nursing facility in King County, Washington.[95]

The *possibility* of presymptomatic transmission of SARS-CoV-2 increases the challenges of COVID-19 containment measures, which are predicated on early detection and isolation of symptomatic persons. The magnitude of this impact is dependent upon the extent and duration of transmissibility while a patient is presymptomatic, *which, to date, have not been clearly established* [all emphases mine].[96]

Scattered throughout the rest of the report were words such as *likely, suggest, suggested, could have occurred, might occur,* etc.

A report from China published in *The* BMJ on April 2, 2020 notes that four-fifths of Covid-19 cases are asymptomatic.[97] Even if there *were* asymptomatic spread, it begs the question how quarantining of healthy individuals would help at all. Tom Jefferson (see footnote 64) calls this four-fifths statistic "very, very important. The sample is small, and more data will become available...let's just say [the results] are generalizable [sic]...then this suggests the virus is

[95] Wei WE, Li Z, Chiew CJ, Yong SE, Toh MP, Lee VJ. Presymptomatic Transmission of SARS-CoV-2 — Singapore, January 23–March 16, 2020. MMWR Morb Mortal Wkly Rep 2020;69:411–415. DOI: http://dx.doi.org/10.15585/mmwr.mm6914e1, p. 411.
[96] Ibid, pp. 414-15.
[97] This would be supported by the evidence I outlined in medical fact #1.

everywhere. If—and I stress, if—the results are representative, then we have to ask, 'what the h-- are we locking down for?'"[98]

Jefferson and his colleague Heneghan write on April 8, 2020: "[There can be] little doubt that the price of lockdown to society and economic paralysis is likely to be paid for generations to come. In the short term economic devastation seems certain, imposing a heavy penalty on us and probably successive generations…Lockdown is going to bankrupt all of us and our descendants and is unlikely at this point to slow or halt viral circulation as the genie is out of the bottle. What the current situation boils down to is this: is the economic meltdown a price worth paying to halt or delay what is already amongst us?"[99]

Professor Yitzhak Ben Israel of Tel Aviv University has plotted the rates of new coronavirus infections in the USA, UK, Sweden, Italy, Israel, Switzerland, France, Germany, and Spain. "The numbers told a shocking story: irrespective of whether the country quarantined like Israel, or went about business as usual like Sweden, coronavirus peaked and subsided in the exact same way…His graphs show that all countries experienced seemingly identical coronavirus infection

---

[98] Day M, Covid-19: four fifths of cases are asymptomatic, China figures indicate, *BMJ* 2020;369:m1375. doi: https://doi.org/10.1136/bmj.m1375 (Published 02 April 2020).
[99] Jefferson & Heneghan, "COVID-19—The Tipping Point," April 8, 2020, at https://www.cebm.net/covid-19/covid-19-the-tipping-point/, accessed ~4/25/2020, re-accessed 9/6/2020. I will address these consequences in chapter 5.

patterns, with the number of infected peaking in the sixth week and rapidly subsiding by the eighth week."[100]

Maria Van Kerkhove, PhD, is an infectious disease epidemiologist and the WHO's Covid-19 technical lead. At a news briefing at the Geneva headquarters on June 8, she stated, "From the data we have, it still seems to be rare that an asymptomatic person actually transmits onward to a secondary individual." She also tweeted, "Comprehensive studies on transmission from asymptomatic individuals are difficult to conduct, but the available evidence from contact tracing reported by Member States suggests that asymptomatically-infected individuals are much less likely to transmit the virus than those who develop symptoms."[101]

In an *Annals of Internal Medicine* study ahead of print, 3,410 close contacts of 391 Covid-19 positive patients in Guangzhou, China were evaluated. The conclusion was that "household contact was the main setting for transmission of SARS-CoV-2 [in contrast to healthcare settings and public transportation], and the risk for transmission of SARS-CoV-2 among close contacts increased with the

---

[100] As reported by Marina Medvin, April 15, 2020, in Townhall. I looked at the Professor's original paper, but it was in Hebrew. This was also reported on April 23, 2020 in the UK's *The Telegraph*, under the title "Coronavirus dies out within 70 days no matter how we tackle it, claims professor."

[101] As reported on Medscape at https://www.medscape.com/viewarticle/931984, accessed 6/9/2020, re-accessed 9/6/2020. Medscape is a physicians' news and CME source. The following day, an editor's note on the site stated: "Since the publication of this story, the WHO has clarified its statement about asymptomatic spread of SARS-CoV-2, calling it a 'misunderstanding.'" Again, do I smell a rat?!

severity of index cases."[102] On May 6, Governor Cuomo of New York reported that "most Covid-19 hospitalizations in New York state [were] from people who were staying home and not venturing much outside."[103] In fact, 66% of new admissions were from people sheltering at home.[104] Cuomo called this fact "shocking." But it's not shocking at all! It's what the data has suggested all along. This highlights the simple wisdom our moms and grandmas told us from little up: *if you're sick, stay home!* Our wise parents and grandparents never told us, *if you're not sick, still stay home, and by all means, put a mask on!* Yet that is the illusion and fear-based paradigm that many parents are currently telling their children.

Put simply, this means you're *very unlikely* to either contract or give Covid-19 in the grocery store; at work; while walking the hallways at church, school, or college; while at the gym; while walking in

---

[102] Luo L, Liu D, Liao X, et al. Contact Settings and Risk for Transmission in 3410 Close Contacts of Patients With COVID-19 in Guangzhou, China : A Prospective Cohort Study [published online ahead of print, 2020 Aug 13]. *Ann Intern Med.* 2020;M20-2671. doi:10.7326/M20-2671. (See footnote #18 in this chapter and footnote #122 In Dr. O'Roark's chapter four.)

[103] As reported at https://www.cnbc.com/2020/05/06/ny-gov-cuomo-says-its-shocking-most-new-coronavirus-hospitalizations-are-people-staying-home.html, accessed 9/6/2020. I had been aware of this statistic for several months prior.

[104] The next highest number in New York was from nursing homes, which accounted for 18% of hospital admissions. Unfortunately, in my state of Pennsylvania, over 2/3 of Covid deaths throughout the state were from nursing homes. This has been widely reported in multiple sources and has been a major pushback to our Governor by state legislators, who have called for the resignation of the PA Department of Health secretary for malpractice and mismanagement.

the park; while singing in a choir[105] or pretty much any other place! Since early April, my clinical gut told me that asymptomatic spread of Covid was a false narrative, and so we put our hypothesis to work in our own office. While we wore masks for about two weeks, we soon discarded them. Since most people with Covid recover uneventfully at home, we kept Covid patients out of the office initially and managed them via phone. More recently, we've brought them in directly to the office like we've done with any other sick patients for several decades. While we've always disinfected exam rooms with medical grade wipes between patients, we did that with extra diligence. We didn't shake hands for a while, but we've been back to that (I've never been a fan of the corona elbow bump) for several months. We haven't social distanced in our office. Anyone who's been in our barn office knows that's not exactly possible, and it's completely impossible to do the work of a physician at six feet! I'm thankful to report we're all doing

---

[105] Choirs and even churches have become paranoid of singing due to the forceful propulsion of aerosol particles. This was highlighted after 45 of 60 choir members attending a choir rehearsal in Washington tested positive (3 weeks after the rehearsal), at least three were hospitalized, and two died. Also, 4 people died of Covid-19 after a choir performance in Amsterdam and two people from a church in Calgary after a service involving singing. It's also true that the average age of the Washington choir was 67 and the two who died were in their 80s (see medical fact #1 above). Most church choirs are comprised of older people. There are far too many health variables involved to extrapolate a policy from these examples for not singing. My wife and I have sung in choirs for many years, and neither of us would be afraid to rejoin normal choir rehearsals today. See https://www.latimes.com/world-nation/story/2020-06-01/coronavirus-choir-singing-cdc-warning and https://people.com/health/washington-choir-members-die-after-rehearsal-amid-coronavirus-spread/, both accessed 9/7/2020.

well, and I know of not a single case of Covid spread from our office. So, thanks be to God, we've proven this in our own office. Yet despite the evidence, so many people in our churches and communities have bought the opposite narrative, and it is to fear that we turn in the next chapter.

CHAPTER 3

Covid-19, Fear, and the Word of God

Daniel O'Roark, DO, FACC

Matthew 10:26-33 (ESV): *²⁶So have no fear of them, for nothing is covered that will not be revealed, or hidden that will not be known. ²⁷What I tell you in the dark, say in the light, and what you hear whispered, proclaim on the housetops. ²⁸And do not fear those who kill the body but cannot kill the soul. Rather fear him who can destroy both soul and body in hell. ²⁹Are not two sparrows sold for a penny? And not one of them will fall to the ground apart from your Father. ³⁰But even the hairs of your head are all numbered. ³¹Fear not, therefore; you are of more value than many sparrows. ³²So everyone who acknowledges me before men, I also will acknowledge before my Father who is in heaven, ³³but whoever denies me before men, I also will deny before my Father who is in heaven.*

Proverbs 1:1-7 (ESV): *¹The proverbs of Solomon, son of David, king of Israel: ²To know wisdom and instruction, to understand words of insight, ³to receive instruction in wise dealing, in righteousness, justice, and equity; ⁴to give prudence to the simple, knowledge and discretion to the youth— ⁵Let the wise hear and increase in learning, and the one who understands obtain guidance, ⁶to understand a proverb and a saying, the words of the wise and their riddles. ⁷The fear of the LORD is the beginning of knowledge; fools despise wisdom and instruction.*

Leviticus 26:36-37 (ESV): [36]...*I will send faintness into their hearts in the lands of their enemies. The sound of a driven leaf shall put them to flight, and they shall flee as one flees from the sword, and they shall fall when none pursues.* [37]*They shall stumble over one another, as if to escape a sword, though none pursues.*

Matthew 6:25-34 (ESV): [25]*"Therefore I tell you, do not be anxious about your life, what you will eat or what you will drink, nor about your body, what you will put on. Is not life more than food, and the body more than clothing?* [26]*Look at the birds of the air: they neither sow nor reap nor gather into barns, and yet your heavenly Father feeds them. Are you not of more value than they?* [27]*And which of you by being anxious can add a single hour to his span of life?* [28]*And why are you anxious about clothing? Consider the lilies of the field, how they grow: they neither toil nor spin,* [29]*yet I tell you, even Solomon in all his glory was not arrayed like one of these.* [30]*But if God so clothes the grass of the field, which today is alive and tomorrow is thrown into the oven, will he not much more clothe you, O you of little faith?* [31]*Therefore do not be anxious, saying, 'What shall we eat?' or 'What shall we drink?' or 'What shall we wear?'* [32]*For the Gentiles seek after all these things, and your heavenly Father knows that you need them all.* [33]*But seek first the kingdom of God and his righteousness, and all these things will be added to you.* [34]*"Therefore do not be anxious about tomorrow, for tomorrow will be anxious for itself. Sufficient for the day is its own trouble."*

A Defining of Terms

Before evaluating the Church's fearful response to the Covid-19 pandemic, it is imperative to establish a foundation of defined terminology. A secular definition of "fear" states:

> **Fear** is an emotion induced by perceived danger or threat, which causes physiological changes and ultimately behavioral changes, such as fleeing, hiding, or freezing from perceived traumatic events. Fear in human beings may occur in response to a certain stimulus occurring in the present, or in anticipation or expectation of a future threat perceived as a risk to oneself. The fear response arises from the perception of danger leading to confrontation with or escape from/avoiding the threat (also known as the fight-or-flight response), which in extreme cases of fear (horror and terror) can be a freeze response or paralysis.

> In humans and animals, fear is modulated by the process of cognition and learning. Thus, fear is judged as rational or appropriate and irrational or inappropriate. An **irrational fear** is called a phobia (emphases added).[1]

---

[1] Wikipedia, *Fear* (https://en.wikipedia.org/wiki/Fear); last edited, 31 August 2020, accessed 9/4/2020.

The "rapid response" of terror-induced fear manifested in the physiologic "fight or flight" response was given by God to Adam at creation[2] and subsequently to all mankind via natural generation.[3]

Virtually all humans have experienced this natural rapid response of physiologic fear. A few examples include the rush to rescue a toddler who has fallen into a swimming pool, the urgency in fleeing a burning building, and clambering frantically to higher ground when the drawback phase[4] of a tsunami is observed.

The response of fear to this sort of catastrophic phenomena is most appropriate and is God-given to aid in the protection and safety of humans.

> God has created self-love in man and wills that we make use of it. The law requires that we love our neighbor as ourselves (Mat 22:39). It is therefore not sinful to fear *deprivation* and *evil*. This fear was inherent in Adam's nature prior to the fall, even though there was no occasion for this fear to arise in him. The Lord Jesus also had such fear (cf. Mat 26:37; Heb 5:7). One may indeed be fearful of death and other discomforts, and *thus also of wild animals and evil men.*[5]

---

[2] Known by way of general revelation.

[3] and is an example of God's "common" Providence.

[4] https://www.sms-tsunami-warning.com/pages/tsunami-drawback#.X1LEP-dJGUk, accessed 9/4/2020.

[5] Wilhelmus À Brakel (1635-1711), *The Fear of God* (A Puritan's Mind,

However, fear is not always conducive to society. Theologically, fear can be either Godly or ungodly. Before exploring the concepts of ungodly fear and its oft present companion anxiety,[6] Wilhelmus À Brakel provides a superb summation of *filial (Godly) fear* and briefly alludes to *servile (ungodly) fear*.[7] He is quoted at length:

> *Filial fear is a holy inclination of the heart, generated by God in the hearts of His children, whereby they, out of reverence for God, take careful pains not to displease God, and earnestly endeavor to please Him in all things. It is a motion of the heart. The noble soul is gifted with emotions, and dependent upon what the objects are, is moved to either joy or sorrow, love or hatred, fear or fearlessness.*

As far as the fear of God is concerned, man is insensitive, hard, and without emotion. "There is no fear of God before their eyes" (Romans 3:18). In regeneration, however, the heart of stone is removed and a heart of flesh is received, which is soft and pliable, and is very readily moved upon beholding God, dependent upon the measure in which God reveals Himself to the soul. If God is perceived as being majestic, a motion immediately arises

---

https://www.apuritansmind.com/the-christian-walk/the-fear-of-god-by-wilhelmus-abrakel/), accessed 9/4/2020.

[6] Most especially as they relate to the coronavirus narrative.

[7] Wilhelmus À Brakel (1635-1711), *The Fear of God.*

within their soul—a motion which is befitting to the creature, in respect to God.

It is a holy motion. Since an unconverted person is in essence nothing but sin, also all that proceeds from him is distorted. The ability to fear is directed toward an erroneous object and is exercised in a disorderly fashion. Believers, however, having been sanctified in principle, are also sanctified as far as their inner motions are concerned. Their fear has a proper object and consequently functions in a holy manner, that is, in faith and love. They are devout and fear God (Act 10:2).

God generates this holy motion. By nature, man is totally unfit for any good work. He finds no delight in God and has no desire to fear the Lord. He may be terrified of God, but he cannot fear Him rightly. However, God enables His own people to fear Him. "I will put My fear in their hearts, that they shall not depart from Me" (Jeremiah 32:40).

The Holy Spirit is therefore called "the Spirit of knowledge and of the fear of the Lord" (Isaiah 11:2).

This filial fear is found in the hearts of God's children. The heart is the seat of all motions—evil as well as good. God has enclosed this precious gift in the hearts of His children, and all the motions relative to fear proceed from the heart. Their fear neither consists in talk, refraining from evil and doing good, nor in the appearance of fear— but rather in truth. The heart, intellect, will, and affections are involved here, and the heart brings forth various deeds which manifest the fear of God. Only God's children truly fear the Lord, and therefore those who have this virtue are called God-fearing people. "...the same man was just and devout" (Luke 2:25); "...devout men" (Acts 2:5); "And devout men carried Stephen to his burial" (Act 8:2).

Filial fear is engendered by reverence for God. God is the object of this fear. "O fear the Lord, you His saints" (Psalm 34:9). God is eminent, glorious, and majestic within Himself—even if there were no creatures. "Yours, O Lord, is the greatness, and the power, and the glory, and the victory, and the majesty" (1 Chr. 29:11). Hereby God is awe-inspiring in and of Himself. With the advent of intelligent creatures who observe the brilliance of His glory, it cannot but be that they have reverence for Him, who is both infinite and majestic.

A natural man does not know God. Therefore, he may be fearful of His judgments, for calamities, and sometimes may acknowledge God to be solemn (although he generally does not progress this far), but he cannot have reverence for Him. That is the privilege and blessedness of believers. A sinful person cannot tolerate God's majesty. He would flee in terror from God, for He is to him a consuming fire.[8] However, in Christ—God is a reconciled Father to His children, and therefore they simultaneously love and revere Him. "Serve the Lord with fear, and rejoice with trembling" (Psalm 2:11) [all emphases added].

A frequent companion of servile fear is anxiety, defined as:

...an emotion characterized by an unpleasant state of inner turmoil, often accompanied by nervous behavior such as pacing back and forth, somatic complaints, and rumination. It is the subjectively unpleasant feelings of dread over anticipated events.

Anxiety is a feeling of uneasiness and worry, usually generalized and unfocused as an overreaction to a situation that is only subjectively seen as menacing. It is often accompanied by muscular tension, restlessness, fatigue and problems in concentration. Anxiety is closely related to fear, which is a response to a real or perceived immediate threat; anxiety involves the expectation of future threat. *People facing anxiety may withdraw from situations which have provoked anxiety in the past* (emphasis added).[9]

---

[8] The natural man exudes what may be termed "servile" fear.

[9] https://en.wikipedia.org/wiki/Anxiety; Last edited on 1 September 2020, accessed 9/4/2020.

The Irrational Association of Servile Fear and Anxiety with Covid-19

During the Covid-19 pandemic, the broader Church often mimicked (in greater or lesser degrees) the fear of the world in their thoughts, words, and deeds with the most regrettable manifestation of this underlying misapprehension being the worldwide near-unanimous suspension of corporate public worship (and along with it the ordinary sanctifying accompaniments of congregational life).

While these are certainly hard words, they are necessary and, Lord willing, stated with and to be received in the spirit of Galatians 6:1-5 and Proverbs 20:30.[10]

As emphasized in Chapter 1 and again quoting Angelo Codevilla from his exceedingly important essay[11] published in the American Mind,[12]

> What history will record as the great COVID scam of 2020 is based on 1) a set of untruths and baseless assertions—often outright lies—about the novel coronavirus and its effects; 2) the production and maintenance of physical fear through a near-monopoly of

---

[10] While physical chastisement is primarily in view here, Godly chastisement in any form is helpful.

[11] Considered a "must read" by the author.

[12] Codevilla, *The Covid Coup* (American Mind, https://americanmind.org/essays/the-covid-coup/?fbclid=IwAR0sC4ZI3yBh-Kium8F6En8C8pCixIDbHt89_zzXQ3RPDNWApGWQ46j0hODE); July 17, 2020, accessed 8/20/2020.

communications to forestall challenges to the U.S. ruling class, led by the Democratic Party, 3) defaulted opposition on the part of most Republicans, thus confirming their status as the ruling class's junior partner. *No default has been greater than that of America's Christian churches—supposedly society's guardians of truth…*

The biggest and most significant default however, has been that of America's Christian churches—all of them—from their hierarchs to their priests, pastors, and ministers. Their complaisance with the lockdowns set aside a truth far more important to human dignity than anything having to do with any physical ailment—the one truth that puts all human power in proper perspective, the truth on which our civilization itself rests: that no human power can manufacture true and false, right and wrong, any more than we can make ourselves, and that, therefore, we are obliged to "render unto Caesar the things that are Caesar's and unto God the things that are God's…"

The churches' agreement to suspend public worship and the distribution of sacraments also contradicted their duty. Until 2020, Christian clergy felt obliged not just to offer public worship to whomever, but also to search out the sick … especially in places where victims of plagues lay between life and death—regardless of consequences. Because surrendering to secular dictates concerning how congregants should behave, even in church cannot be

114

justified in Christian terms *it would not have crossed previous generations of churchmen's minds.*

Had this generation of church leaders simply practiced their faith, even by merely keeping silent about the ruling class's claims about COVID-19 rather than ignorantly, submissively endorsing them, they would have preserved their intellectual and moral credit to help the general population to deal with the growing realization that they had been duped (all emphases added).

Scripture is explicit in its condemnation of anxiety and irrational, servile fear amongst the people of God. Matthew 6:25-34 warns us to avoid this type of emotional state as it reflects a lack of trust in the absolute sovereignty of God in all that occurs in the created universe—including the minute details of our lives.

The presence of ungodly fear in the Church is an *implicit* [13] *rejection of the biblical truth that the day, time, and means of our death have all been determined by the absolute, irrevocable and secret decree of God in eternity past.* [14] Some of us may be foreordained to die as a result of SARS-CoV-2 infection, but for the majority it will be something else that ushers us into the eternal state.

---

[13] albeit often subconsciously held.

[14] This is in no way to be interpreted as endorsing a cavalier, callous, and/or reckless attitude toward various life risks. Certainly, God is not to be tempted. What is argued for here is a measured, rational, and balanced approach to risk assessment.

It is completely understandable that the unregenerate might wallow in servile and irrational fears. Having adopted a materialistic, evolutionary, atheistic (or unitarian) mindset, they are pushed into a contradictory belief system that desires the preservation of life regardless of cost as "this life is all we have."[15]

The Church's Complicity in Servile Fear & Anxiety

The final part of this chapter considers several ways the Church exhibited irrational fear and anxiety throughout the world in the Covid-19 pandemic.[16]

In the a priori acceptance of the mainstream media/CDC/WHO Covid-19 pandemic narrative.

Given the draconian and high stakes content of what was explicitly asserted as absolutely necessary for the "survival of humanity," should not Christians simply have asked, "Is this true?"

---

[15] Of course, this is contradictory and irrational on their part given their absolute love of death in other areas of life (unrepentant, habitual sin, suicide, abortion on demand, infanticide, etc. – Proverbs 8:35-36).

[16] A number of these precepts have been elucidated in my chapter 4 on sphere sovereignty.

In the suspension of public worship.

Disruptions to public worship occurred even though most everyone (had they dared trusting their senses) could see that very few were actually dying or being hospitalized from the virus! Data shows that Covid-19 possesses an infection fatality rate (IFR) across all age groups of about 0.2%;[17] this is slightly higher than influenza fatality rates, yet note that these statistics fall almost exclusively in the domain of the chronically and seriously ill—most of whom are/were extremely aged.

The overwhelming majority of congregants are in very low (ages 0-14, virtually no mortality)[18] and low (ages 15-64) risk groups with the latter group having a 3.6 per 100,000 mortality rate.[19] For these persons, Covid-19 poses a death rate equivalent to or slightly lower than the yearly 0.1% influenza death risk.

The Covid-19 morbidity and mortality statistics are often interpreted without context—obviously yielding incorrect conclusions. Currently, the United States population is estimated at 331

---

[17] Anthony Fauci et. al. *Covid-19 — Navigating the Uncharted* (New England Journal of Medicine; February 28, 2020; online at https://www.nejm.org/doi/full/10.1056/NEJMe2002387), accessed 8/22/2020.

[18] Given these realities, why were church nurseries, Sunday Schools, and other ministries for children suspended?

[19] Overall, all-cause mortality for this population is 335 per 100,000. David Stockman, *The Three Nations of Covid and a Windbag Named Fauci* (Lew Rockwell.com, https://www.lewrockwell.com/2020/05/david-stockman/the-three-nations-of-covid-and-a-windbag-named-fauci/) May 2, 2020, accessed 8/29/2020.

million with about 2.8 million annual deaths.[20] The world population is just shy of 8 billion with about 60 million yearly expires.[21] Upon calculation (and accepting the overinflated death statistics[22] as accurate [which we do not]), Covid-19 will be responsible for about 6% of all deaths in the U.S. and worldwide about 1.1% (in 2020). Here *we hardly see a disease that warrants "plague-designated status."*

Within the framework of available data, should not Christians and their earthly Shepherds have questioned the culture-destroying lock-downs and physical distancing measures for *this* virus when we have *never* done the same for the roughly equivalent and *yearly* influenza pandemics?

[20] Worldometer, *Countries in the world by population (2020)* (https://www.worldometers.info/world-population/population-by-country/); September 2020 (accessed 9/5/2020).

[21] Hannah Ritchie, *How many people die and how many are born each year?* (Our World in Data, https://ourworldindata.org/births-and-deaths); September 19, 2019, accessed 9/5/2020.

[22] CDC/WHO estimates about 170,000 SARS-Cov-2 fatalities in the USA and 700,000 worldwide.

In the acceptance of ineffective,[23, 24, 25] *dehumanizing mask*[26] *and social distancing mandates.*[27]

Too many elders, without Scriptural warrant, made these measures a *condition* for church attendance. This egregious error has led church councils, apparently unwittingly so, to be "respecters of persons" (contra James 2:1-13) as the opinions of the Covid-19 "believers" are given precedence over the beliefs of the "skeptics." An item of apparel (the mask) has become, in many congregations, a *compulsory* "ticket" for access to the preached Word and Sacraments.

---

[23] Desai & Mehrotra, "Medical Masks," *JAMA.* 2020;323(15):1517-1518. doi:10.1001/jama.2020.2331, published March 4, 2020.

[24] Michael Klompas, Charles Morris, et. al., *Universal Masking in Hospitals in the Covid-19 Era* (New England Journal of Medicine, https://www.nejm.org/doi/full/10.1056/NEJMp2006372); April 1, 2020, accessed 9/8/2020.

[25] Tom Jefferson, Chris Del Mar, et. al., *Physical interventions to interrupt or reduce the spread of respiratory viruses* (Cochrane Library, https://www.ncbi.nlm.nih.gov/pmc/articles/PMC6993921/); July 6, 2011, accessed 9/8/2020.

[26] Stephen Halbrook, *Face Binding: Masks as the New Foot Binding* (Vaccines and Christianity, https://www.vaccinesandchristianity.org/2020/08/22/face-binding-masks-as-the-new-foot-binding/); August 22, 2020 (accessed 9/5/2020).

[27] Stephen Halbrook, Why Churches must Oppose Mandated Social Distancing: it's not as Benign as you Think (Vaccines and Christianity, https://www.vaccinesandchristianity.org/2020/05/15/dangers-of-social-distancing-to-the-church/); May 15, 2020, accessed 9/5/2020.

Colossians 2:20-22 (ESV): *²⁰If with Christ you died to the elemental spirits of the world, why, as if you were still alive in the world, do you submit to regulations—²¹ "Do not handle, Do not taste, Do not touch" ²² (referring to things that all perish as they are used)—according to human precepts and teachings?*

More distressing, and in violation of the 9th commandment to not bear false witness, is the explicit notion that all the apparently healthy *must* be considered occult disease bearers[28] and are therefore necessarily "unclean"—especially in the absence of a facemask. This falsity has led to physical aversion amongst various image bearers of God engendered by disease-suspicion towards one another.

In the spiritually unhealthy preoccupation with "health and safety as a top congregational priority."[29]

This is expressed by a "germaphobia"[30] which brings to light an implicit, irrational fear of sickness and death amongst some of God's people.

---

[28] with no evidence of any kind required.

[29] a manifestly unbiblical concept.

[30] *In mimicry of the world,* many churches have removed the hymn books, eliminated paper bulletins, maniacally spray the pews with disinfectants, rope off pews, prohibit the use of water fountains, etc.

In the unwitting promotion of a narrative based upon and bathed in a sea of malpresentations; incompetence; lies; deceit; massive contradictions; medical, apologetical, epistemological, and common-sense (logical) errors; conflicts of interest and more.

Notwithstanding their very own observations, many Christians have allowed *"the sound of a driven leaf [to] put them to flight."* Covid-19 is real and has indeed caused significant sickness and even death but, nevertheless, represents a pandemic that is not all that extraordinary in world history. ***Despite this fact, the Church in many places has taken up extreme and authoritarian responses to the pandemic markedly out of proportion to its actual threat.***

It should be patently manifest that the Church of the Lord Jesus Christ should not only strenuously avoid participating in such paradigms of darkness but make vigorous effort to shine the brilliant light of God's truth on them and other dubious schemes.

Prayer as an Antidote to Fear and Anxiety

Matthew 26:36-39 (ESV): [36]*Then Jesus went with them to a place called Gethsemane, and he said to his disciples, "Sit here, while I go over there and pray." *[37]* And taking with him Peter and the two sons of Zebedee, he began to be sorrowful and troubled. *[38]*Then he said to them, "My soul is very sorrowful, even to death; remain here, and watch with me." *[39]*And going a* *little farther he fell on his face and prayed, saying, "My Father, if it be pos-sible, let this cup pass from me; nevertheless, not as I will, but as you will."*

Luke 22:41-44 (ESV): [41]*And he withdrew from them about a stone's throw, and knelt down and prayed,* [42]*saying, "Father, if you are willing, remove this cup from me. Nevertheless, not my will, but yours, be done."* [43]*And there appeared to him an angel from heaven, strengthening him.* [44]*And being in agony he prayed more earnestly; and his sweat became like great drops of blood falling down to the ground.*

Mark 14:32-36 (ESV): [32]*And they went to a place called Gethsemane. And he said to his disciples, "Sit here while I pray."* [33]*And he took with him Peter and James and John, and began to be greatly distressed and troubled.* [34]*And he said to them, "My soul is very sorrowful, even to death. Remain here and watch."* [35]*And going a little farther, he fell on the ground and prayed that, if it were possible, the hour might pass from him.* [36]*And he said, "Abba, Father, all things are possible for you. Remove this cup from me. Yet not what I will, but what you will."*

Psalm 91:1-16 (ESV): [1]*He who dwells in the shelter of the Most High will abide in the shadow of the Almighty.* [2]*I will say to the LORD, "My refuge and my fortress, my God, in whom I trust."* [3]*For he will deliver you from the snare of the fowler and from the deadly pestilence.* [4]*He will cover you with his pinions, and under his wings you will find refuge; his faithfulness is a shield and buckler.* [5]*You will not fear the terror of the night, nor the arrow that flies by day,* [6]*nor the pestilence that stalks in darkness, nor the* *destruction that wastes at noonday. ⁷A thousand may fall at your side, ten thousand at your right hand, but it will not come near you. ⁸You will only look with your eyes and see the recompense of the wicked. ⁹Because you have made the LORD your dwelling place—the Most High, who is my refuge— ¹⁰no evil shall be allowed to befall you, no plague come near your tent. ¹¹For he will command his angels concerning you to guard you in all your ways. ¹²On their hands they will bear you up, lest you strike your foot against a stone. ¹³You will tread on the lion and the adder; the young lion and the serpent you will trample underfoot. ¹⁴"Because he holds fast to me in love, I will deliver him; I will protect him, because he knows my name. ¹⁵When he calls to me, I will answer him; I will be with him in trouble; I will rescue him and honor him. ¹⁶With long life I will satisfy him and show him my salvation."*

Psalm 34:4 (ESV): *I sought the LORD, and he answered me and delivered me from all my fears.*

Psalm 23:4 (ESV): *Even though I walk through the valley of the shadow of death, I will fear no evil, for you are with me; your rod and your staff, they comfort me.*

Isaiah 38:1-8 (ESV): *¹In those days Hezekiah became sick and was at the point of death. And Isaiah the prophet the son of Amoz came to him, and said to him, "Thus says the LORD: Set your house in order, for you shall die, you shall not recover." ²Then Hezekiah turned his face to the wall and prayed to the LORD, ³and said, "Please, O LORD, remember how I have* *walked before you in faithfulness and with a whole heart, and have done what is good in your sight." And Hezekiah wept bitterly.* ⁴*Then the word of the LORD came to Isaiah:* ⁵*"Go and say to Hezekiah, Thus says the LORD, the God of David your father: I have heard your prayer; I have seen your tears. Behold, I will add fifteen years to your life.* ⁶*I will deliver you and this city out of the hand of the king of Assyria, and will defend this city.* ⁷*"This shall be the sign to you from the LORD, that the LORD will do this thing that he has promised:* ⁸*Behold, I will make the shadow cast by the declining sun on the dial of Ahaz turn back ten steps." So the sun turned back on the dial the ten steps by which it had declined.*

3 John 1:2 (ESV): *The elder to the beloved Gaius, whom I love in truth. 2 Beloved, I pray that all may go well with you and that you may be in good health, as it goes well with your soul.*

Philippians 4:6-7 (ESV): ⁶*Do not be anxious about anything, but in everything by prayer and supplication with thanksgiving let your requests be made known to God.* ⁷*And the peace of God, which surpasses all understanding, will guard your hearts and your minds in Christ Jesus.*

1 Peter 5:6-8 (ESV): ⁶*Humble yourselves, therefore, under the mighty hand of God so that at the proper time he may exalt you,* ⁷*casting all your anxieties on him, because he cares for you.* ⁸*Be sober-minded; be watchful. Your adversary the devil prowls around like a roaring lion, seeking someone to devour.*

Romans 8:26-28 (ESV): *[26]Likewise, the Spirit helps us in our weakness. For we do not know what to pray for as we ought, but the Spirit himself intercedes for us with groanings too deep for words. [27]And he who searches hearts knows what is the mind of the Spirit, because the Spirit intercedes for the saints according to the will of God. [28]And we know that for those who love God all things work together for good, for those who are called according to his purpose.*

Christ Has Won Victory Over Death

1 Corinthians 15:20-28 (ESV): *[20]But in fact, Christ has been raised from the dead, the first fruits of those who have fallen asleep. [21]For as by a man came death, by a man has come also the resurrection of the dead. [22]For as in Adam all die, so also in Christ shall all be made alive. [23]But each in his own order: Christ the first fruits, then at his coming those who belong to Christ. [24]Then comes the end, when he delivers the kingdom to God the Father after destroying every rule and every authority and power. [25]For he must reign until he has put all his enemies under his feet. [26]The last enemy to be destroyed is death. [27]For "God has put all things in subjection under his feet." But when it says, "all things are put in subjection," it is plain that he is excepted who put all things in subjection under him. [28]When all things are subjected to him, then the Son himself will also be subjected to him who put all things in subjection under him, that God may be all in all.*

1 Corinthians 15:51-58 (ESV): *[51]Behold! I tell you a mystery. We shall not all sleep, but we shall all be changed, [52]in a moment, in the twinkling* *of an eye, at the last trumpet. For the trumpet will sound, and the dead will be raised imperishable, and we shall be changed. [53] For this perishable body must put on the imperishable, and this mortal body must put on immortality. [54] When the perishable puts on the imperishable, and the mortal puts on immortality, then shall come to pass the saying that is written:*

"Death is swallowed up in victory."
[55] "O death, where is your victory?
O death, where is your sting?"

[56] The sting of death is sin, and the power of sin is the law. [57] But thanks be to God, who gives us the victory through our Lord Jesus Christ.

[58] Therefore, my beloved brothers, be steadfast, immovable, always abounding in the work of the Lord, knowing that in the Lord your labor is not in vain.

A filial fear of death is righteous and appropriate. An irrational fear of dying amongst professing Christians is not. True believers are temporally and eternally safe in Christ. Persecutions and a multitude of other earthly trials and tribulations may come but the Christian is to "hide in the cleft of the Rock," that Rock being Christ.

The expressions of J.I. Packer capture nicely the intent of the teachings of Scripture:

MORTALITY:
CHRISTIANS NEED NOT FEAR DEATH
by J.I. Packer[31]

For to me, to live is Christ and to die is gain. If I am to go on living in the body, this will mean fruitful labor for me. Yet what shall I choose? I do not know! I am torn between the two: I desire to depart and be with Christ, which is better by far; but it is more necessary for you that I remain in the body. Philippians 1:21-24

We do not know how humans would have left this world had there been no Fall; some doubt whether they ever would have done so. But as it is, the separation of body and soul through bodily death, which is both sin's fruit and God's judgment (Gen. 2:17; 3:19, 22; Rom. 5:12; 8:10; 1 Cor. 15:21), is one of life's certainties. This separating of the soul (person) from the body is a sign and emblem of the spiritual separation from God that first brought about physical death (Gen. 2:17; 5:5) and that will be deepened after death for those who leave this world without Christ. Naturally, therefore, death appears as an enemy (1 Cor. 15:26) and a terror (Heb. 2:15).

For Christians the terror of physical death is abolished, though the unpleasantness of dying remains. Jesus, their

---

[31] J.I. Packer, *Mortality: Christians Need Not Fear Death* (excerpted from Concise Theology: A Guide to Historic Christian Beliefs, https://www.monergism.com/thethreshold/articles/onsite/packer/death.html); 2008, accessed 9/8/2020.

risen Savior, has himself passed through a more traumatic death than any Christian will ever have to face, and he now lives to support his servants as they move out of this world to the place he has prepared for them in the next world (John 14:2-3). Christians should view their own forthcoming death as an appointment in Jesus' calendar, which he will faithfully keep. Paul could say, "For to me, to live is Christ and to die is gain.... I desire to depart and be with Christ, which is better by far" (Phil. 1:21, 23), since "away from the body" will mean "at home with the Lord" (2 Cor. 5:8) ...

... Death is decisive for destiny. After death there is no possibility of salvation for the lost (Luke 16:26)—from then on both the godly and the ungodly reap what they sowed in this life (Gal. 6:7-8).

Death is gain for believers (Phil. 1:21) because after death they are closer to Christ. But disembodiment, as such, is not gain; bodies are for expression and experience, and to be without a body is to be limited, indeed impoverished. This is why Paul wants to be "clothed" with his resurrection body (i.e., re-embodied) rather than be "unclothed" (i.e., disembodied, 2 Cor. 5:1-4). To be resurrected for the life of heaven is the true Christian hope. As life in the "intermediate" or "interim" state between death and resurrection is better than the life in this world that preceded it, so the life of resurrection will be better still. It will, in fact, be best. And this is what God has in store for all his children (2 Cor. 5:4-5; Phil. 3:20-21). Hallelujah!

CONCLUSIONS

Jesus lives, and so shall I. Death! Thy sting is gone forever!
He who deigned for me to die, Lives, the bands of death to sever.
He shall raise me from the dust: Jesus is my Hope and Trust.[32]

(Amen)

Who trusts in God, a strong abode in heaven and earth possesses;
Who looks in love to Christ above, No fear his heart oppresses.
In thee alone, dear Lord, we own sweet hope and consolation;
Until we stand at Thy right hand, Through Jesus' saving merit.[33]

(Amen)

---

[32] Christian F. Gellert, *Hymn 596, The Trinity Hymnal* (Philadelphia, Pa., The Orthodox Presbyterian Church); 1961.

[33] Joachim Magdeburg, *Hymn 558, The Trinity Hymnal* (Philadelphia, Pa., The Orthodox Presbyterian Church); 1961.

CHAPTER 4

The Necessity and Vital Importance of Jurisdictionalism (Sphere Sovereignty) to Christian and Societal Liberty: The Biblical Limitations of Civil and Ecclesiastical Power

Daniel O'Roark, DO, FACC

Romans 13:1-7 (ESV): *¹Let every person be subject to the governing authorities. For there is no authority except from God, and those that exist have been instituted by God. ²Therefore whoever resists the authorities resists what God has appointed, and those who resist will incur judgment. ³For rulers are not a terror to good conduct, but to bad. Would you have no fear of the one who is in authority? Then do what is good, and you will receive his approval, ⁴for he is God's servant for your good. But if you do wrong, be afraid, for he does not bear the sword in vain. For he is the servant of God, an avenger who carries out God's wrath on the wrongdoer. ⁵Therefore one must be in subjection, not only to avoid God's wrath but also for the sake of conscience. ⁶For because of this you also pay taxes, for the authorities are ministers of God, attending to this very thing. ⁷Pay to all what is owed to them: taxes to whom taxes are owed, revenue to whom revenue is owed, respect to whom respect is owed, honor to whom honor is owed.*

Hebrews 13:17 (ESV): *Obey your leaders and submit to them, for they are keeping watch over your souls, as those who will have to give an account. Let them do this with joy and not with groaning, for that would be of no advantage to you.*

Acts 5:25-29 (ESV): *25And someone came and told them, "Look! The men whom you put in prison are standing in the temple and teaching the people." 26Then the captain with the officers went and brought them, but not by force, for they were afraid of being stoned by the people. 27And when they had brought them, they set them before the council. And the high priest questioned them, 28saying, "We strictly charged you not to teach in this name, yet here you have filled Jerusalem with your teaching, and you intend to bring this man's blood upon us." 29But Peter and the apostles answered, "We must obey God rather than men.*

Acts 17:10-11 (ESV): *10The brothers immediately sent Paul and Silas away by night to Berea, and when they arrived, they went into the Jewish synagogue. 11Now these Jews were more noble than those in Thessalonica; they received the word with all eagerness, examining the Scriptures daily to see if these things were so.*

The "great" Coronavirus (SARS-CoV-2[1] [Covid-19]) pandemic of 2020 has caused much grief and misery around the world but most especially in these United States. Interestingly, and as reviewed elsewhere in this volume, it did so *not primarily* by way of unprecedented and unique morbidity and mortality[2]—indeed, it has not been half as bad[3] as the Asian (1957) and Hong Kong influenza (1968/69) pandemics of the past—*but in the civil and ecclesiastical responses to it.*

A careful examination of Scripture, the Westminster Standards[4] (the subordinate confessional statements of many Presbyterians bodies), and the Presbyterian Church in America (PCA)[5] Book of Church Order (BCO)[6,7] will demonstrate that a plethora of civil

---

[1] The presumptive viral etiology of the Covid-19 syndrome.

[2] Each of the Asian and Hong Kong influenza pandemics were estimated to have killed between 1.2 to 4 million persons worldwide; Covid-19, taking the global mortality data at face value, has (as of 8/12/2020) taken the lives of about 700,000.

[3] This statement is in no way intended to minimize or make light of the impact of Covid-19 on individuals and families which has included serious illness, hospitalizations and deaths. Nevertheless, by nature, the fields of epidemiology and vital statistics are necessarily "matter of fact" and emotionless in their presentation. Who was sick or injured? Why? And, did the afflicted die as a result of the illness/injury or suffer serious morbidity?

[4] *Westminster Confession of Faith* (WCF) (http://clearnotesongbook.com/confessions/westminster-confession-faith-1647); 1647, accessed 8/12/2020.

[5] The denominational affiliation of the authors.

[6] *PCA Book of Church Order (BCO)* (https://www.pcaac.org/wp-content/uploads/2019/10/BCO-2019-with-bookmarks-for-website-1.pdf); 2019, accessed 8/13/2020.

[7] Along with Scripture and the Westminster Standards, the BCO is a part of the PCA Constitution.

magistrates and church officers oft exceeded the authority given to them by God during the pandemic.

As a consequence of the latter, the "peace and purity"[8] of the church has been frequently disrupted.

The peace of the church has been disturbed by the unwarranted suspension of *gathered* public worship[9] thereby hindering believers' access to the in-person preaching of Word of God and the administration of the sacraments.[10] Many congregations have divided more or less into several camps: Covid-19 skeptics, the non-skeptics, and a larger group of the "significantly uncertain." Some Christian families have restricted visitation amongst one another so as to "prevent the spread" thereby leading to "disease suspicion" and social isolation.

Church purity has been affected by erroneous applications of biblical law, an improper understanding of church-state relations,[11] and a defective interpretation and application of the ever

---

[8] These terms refer to the preservation of (a) Christian unity (peace) within the local and broader assemblies of the church and (b) pure doctrine (purity) both to be driven by an unwavering commitment to the inerrant, infallible Word of God.

[9] While extraordinarily useful for evangelism of the unchurched and of great benefit for those *providentially hindered* from attending public worship services, it must be emphatically declared that the viewing of recorded or "live" streamed church services *does not* meet the biblical requirement to "physically gather" with God's people on the Lord's Day. In other words, one "does not go to church" via livestream.

[10] As well as other sanctifying accompaniments of congregational life: evangelism including campus, nursing home and prison ministries; reception of new members; ordination vows; church discipline; marriage and funeral ceremonies; in-person prayer meetings, etc.

[11] Resulting from a faulty exegesis of Romans 13:1-7 and 1 Peter 2:13–17.

important "Love Thy Neighbor" precept as it applies to contagious illness and public health. As peace and purity are inseparable constructs, a disruption of purity also upsets community peace.

When congregations did ultimately return to public worship, it was often in the context of a fear based ("Sickness Cult") paradigm of excessive social distancing measures, mask mandates, and explicit commands to avoid ordinary human interaction such as hugs, handshakes, and speaking with one another in the pews.

The Biblical Limitations of Civil Power

The doctrine of *Sphere Sovereignty* is structured by four God-ordained governing domains on this earth: the *individual* (self-government), *family*, *church*, and *state* (civil magistrate). While distinct from one another (and with some unavoidable overlap, e.g. the child as an individual while at the same time being under authority of family), these spheres of jurisdiction are *always and ultimately* operative under the precepts of the triune God and His Law-Word *alone*.

When these several governments (most often the state) act in such a way as to "get out of their lanes" (so to speak), tyranny is often the result.

Recalling the formulations of Abraham Kuyper,[12] Joe Boot states:

---

[12] Abraham Kuyper (1837–1920) was a Dutch Calvinistic Christian, university founder, and politician. In 1874 he was elected to his nation's lower house of Parliament and served there

135

The basic creational principle at work here is what Abraham Kuyper called *Sphere Sovereignty* (Gen. 2:21-25; 9:5-6; 1 Sam. 13:10-14; 1 Kgs. 21:1-16; Mark 12:13-17; John 19:5-12; Acts 5:22-32; Col. 1:15-20; Eph. 1:20-23; 1 Tim. 3:14-16; Rev. 1:5) There are varied spheres of life within human society, i.e. the family, church, business, educational institutions, the arts and so forth, which do not *owe their existence* to the state, nor do they *derive their internal sphere of law* from the state. These spheres of life must obey the authority of God and His Word over them. They are not subservient to the state, nor do they relate to the state in parts-to-whole fashion as though they were lesser 'parts' of the state. As such the state has no right to overreach and intrude into them.

This principle helps us distinguish a *just state* from an absolutist *power state*. A just state will recognize a variety of *spheres of law* within society including public law, civil private law and non-civil private law. Public law concerns the constitution, penal law and laws of criminal procedure as well as administrative law – these are meant to guarantee our political freedoms. Common law, or civil private law, exists to guarantee our freedom of thought and expression, association and so forth, making sure that in social entities

until 1877 after which he left politics for a time and founded the Free University of Amsterdam. In 1901, Kuyper returned to politics as the Prime Minister of the Netherlands, a post he held until 1905.

we are on an equal footing with others. Critically, non-civil private law concerns the existence and freedom of non-political spheres of law, like the church. The civil magistrate cannot command or interpret the proper nature of Christian worship, for example, because this is non-civil private law and outside of the state's competency.[13]

And similarly, as remarked by Larry Farlow,

All governments claim a degree of sovereignty over their people. The question, Kuyper says, is from what source does that authority flow? The answer is, that authority flows from God alone:

In whatever form this authority may reveal itself, man never possesses power over his fellow-man in any other way than by an authority which descends upon him from the majesty of God.

--- Kuyper, Abraham. Lectures on Calvinism (p. 77). Eerdmans Publishing Co – A. Kindle Edition.

This is as opposed to what Kuyper calls 'Popular-sovereignty' and 'State-sovereignty' ...

---

[13] Joe Boot, *Freedom, the Church and State Absolutism* (Ezra Institute, https://www.ezrainstitute.ca/resource-library/articles/freedom-the-church-and-state-absolutism/); July 15, 2020, accessed 8/23/2020.

… Popular-sovereignty believes ultimate power is vested with the people. This is the model on which the French Revolution was built, pure democracy. On the other hand, you have states such as Nazi Germany and, currently, North Korea, where the state is sovereign over all things. Interestingly, Kuyper, when writing this in 1898, identified the German Empire as an example of this kind of government. Clearly, Germany's National Socialism of the 1930s didn't appear from nowhere but grew up from already plowed soil. A sober warning.

In the first of these models, *the individual is subservient to the tyranny of the majority, in the second the state becomes an almost mythical being to whom all must swear allegiance.* **In neither model are the rights of the individual and the freedom of the church protected because in neither model are any constraints placed on the sovereign whether that is the majority of the voters** ["*democracy,*" author's note, DO] **or a dictator** [emphasis added].[14]

---

[14] Larry Farlow, *Kuyper's Sovereignty in the Sphere of Society* (https://forgodsfame.org/2018/02/13/kuypers-sovereignty-in-the-sphere-of-society/); February 2018, accessed 8/23/2020. "Under sovereignty of the sphere, each institution, the government, the church, the family, the arts, business, etc. is answerable to God within the sphere of their responsibility and function. No sphere owes its existence to any of the others but operates independently under God's sovereignty: *In a Calvinistic sense we understand hereby, that the family, the business, science, art and so forth are all social spheres, which do not owe their existence to the state, and which do not derive the law of their life from the superiority of the state, but obey a high authority within their own bosom; an authority which rules, by the grace of God, just as the*

In light of these considerations, it cannot be overemphasized that no man, woman, or child owes any other man, woman, or child blind and unfettered obedience but must be strictly guided in conduct by God's word alone.

When commanded by a superior[15] to do something required by God's law, we *must do it* as it is *always* our duty—whether superiors necessitate it or not. On the other hand, when we are directed by a superior to do something forbidden by God's Law, *we must disobey* as God and God alone is the Lord of conscience (WCF Chapter 20, especially 20.2).[16]

Far too many in the Presbyterian and Reformed communities have accentuated *only* the duties of inferiors towards superiors[17] while virtually neglecting the *duties owed* by superiors *to* their inferiors (Westminster Larger Catechism (LC), Questions 129-130). The following four concepts help establish a biblical framework.

---

sovereignty of the State does -- Kuyper, Abraham. Lectures on Calvinism (p. 82). Eerdmans Publishing Co – A. Kindle Edition.'"

[15] Be it an employer, mother or father, husband, civil magistrate, church session or council or other derived authority figures.

[16] This incredibly important section of the WCF will be explored more fully later in this chapter.

[17] Especially in the context of church-state relations and the relationship of the Office of Believer to the Office of Civil Magistracy.

First, there absolutely exists a *biblical* separation of church and state[18] but the *myth* widely promulgated now is that the state (civil magistracy or statecraft) is independent of and separated from the Law of God (contra Psalm 2).

Second, the moral Law of God, as summarized by the Ten Commandments, applies to all men everywhere *in their respective spheres of jurisdiction.*[19] Therefore, civil magistrates, in their capacity as magistrates, are duty-bound to pattern their obligations by special revelation (Scripture) *alone.*[20, 21]

Third, as all humans have a duty to repent and by faith receive Christ as He is offered in the Gospel (Acts 17:30), the civil magistrate

---

[18] George Gillespie, *Aaron's Rod Blossoming* (https://archive.org/details/aablossom00gill/page/n3/mode/2up); Published 1646, accessed 8/12/2020.

[19] See *Westminster Confession of Faith* [WCF] 19.2 with scripture proofs* / 19.5* and the *Westminster Larger Catechism* [LC] Q/A 91* / 93-98*, (http://clearnotesongbook.com/confessions/westminster-larger-catechism-1646); 1646, accessed 8/12/2020.

[20] Within and outside the visible church, many erroneously appeal to natural law (NL) (usually coupled with human reason) as the ultimate source of authority for the civil magistrate. NL, written by the Lord on the hearts of all men beginning with pre-lapsarian Adam, is the source of conscience (Romans 2:12-16) and is essentially equivalent to the Ten Commandments (the *summary* of the moral law). Nevertheless, since the fall of Adam, NL is no longer a *reliable* guide for orthodox doctrine and conduct as men have become totally depraved as a consequence of original sin (all people are thoroughly sinful in thought, word and deed, albeit to varying degrees) and suppress the truths of God in unrighteousness (Romans 1:18-32). The Bible alone is to be our sole authority (2 Timothy 3:16-17, WCF 1.6 and 1.10) and is, therefore, the only reliable and authoritative guide for individuals, families, church leaders and civil magistrates regarding "right doctrine and deeds".

[21] For a succinct but thorough treatment of Natural Law, see Phillip G. Kayser, *The Flaw of Natural Law* (Omaha, NE. Biblical Blueprints [www.biblicalblueprints.org]); 2009.

likewise is *expected by God* to be a Christian. (Psalm 2, most especially vss. 10-12).[22]

Fourth, the office of civil magistrate is ordained by God. He is the Lord's minister – a servant (Romans 13:1-7). This text is prescriptive or normative[23] as to how the *righteous magistrate* carries out his callings before God. It is a template for the duties, boundaries, and conduct of all civil magistrates whether they be regenerate or not.

> It then belongs to princes to know how far they may extend their authority, and to subjects in what they may obey them, lest the one encroaching on that jurisdiction, which no way belongs to them, and the others obeying him which commands further than he ought, they be both chastised, when they shall give an account thereof before another judge. Now the end and scope of the question propounded, whereof the Holy Scripture shall principally give the resolution, is that which follows. The question is, if subjects be bound to obey kings, in case they command that which is against the law of God: that is to say, to which of the two (God or king) must we rather obey, when the question shall be resolved concerning the king, to whom is attributed

---

[22] Exodus 18:21; 2 Samuel 23:3; 2 Chronicles 19:4-10

[23] A normative or prescriptive Scripture text describes how things *ought* to be not necessarily how they actually are. By contrast, a descriptive text portrays how things *are*, not necessarily how they ought to be. Some biblical texts are both normative and descriptive and often one must compare Scripture with Scripture to elucidate the full and proper meaning of any particular passage (WCF 1.7).

absolute power, that concerning other magistrates shall be also determined.

First, the Holy Scripture does teach that God reigns by his own proper authority, and kings by derivation. God from himself, kings from God, that God has a jurisdiction proper, kings are his delegates. It follows then, that the jurisdiction of God has no limits, that of kings bounded, that the power of God is infinite, that of kings confined, that the kingdom of God extends itself to all places, that of kings is restrained within the confines of certain countries. In like manner God had created of nothing both heaven and earth; wherefore by good right He is lord, and true proprietor, both of the one and the other. All the inhabitants of the earth hold of Him that which they have, and are but His tenants and farmers; all the princes and governors of the world are His stipendiaries and vassals, and are bound to take and acknowledge their investitures from Him. Briefly, God alone is the owner and lord, and all men of what degree or quality so ever they be, are His servants, farmers, officers and vassals, and owe account and acknowledgement to Him, according to that which He has committed to their dispensation; the higher their place is, the greater their account must be, and according to the ranks whereunto God has raised them, must they make their reckoning before His divine majesty, which the Holy Scriptures teach in infinite places, and all the faithful, yea, and the wisest among the heathen have ever acknowledged.[24]

And, as observed by Joe Boot,

> In Romans 13, Paul specifically and explicitly places *all authority* under God, including civil government, as a sphere of power and authority instituted by Him alone. The apostle's exhortation against resisting God's order in temporal authority, assumes that to do so resists *God's command* (v. 2). What is at issue here is man's propensity to resist *God's* ordinances and commands. Clearly, we cannot selectively obey God's commands at our convenience—including recognizing the legitimacy of temporal authority. This being the case, if the state presumes to forbid what God commands, or commands what God forbids, the state has moved beyond its sphere of authority, and those who obey God must at that point resist such arrogant presumption. This is clear from what follows when Paul shows that the civil authority is God's servant – that is literally God's *deacon* (v. 4). The apostle explains that this means being a terror

---

[24] Stephen Junius Brutus (Pseudonym thought to be Hubert Languet or Philippe de Mornay), A Defense of Liberty Against Tyrants (Excerpts Vindiciae contra Tyrannos: A Defence of Liberty against Tyrants, OR, Of the Lawful Power of the Prince over the People and of the People over the Prince. A Treatise written in Latin and French by Junius Brutus, and Translated out of both into English. London: Richard Baldwin. http://www.nlnrac.org/classical/late-medieval-transformations/documents/defense); 1689, accessed 9/15/2020.

to bad conduct and approving of good conduct, bearing the sword to avenge those that do wrong (vv. 3-4). *But if the state becomes a terror to those who do good and rewards those that do evil, it is again in flagrant violation of God's command and ordinance, and Christians have at that point a duty to resist an authority that has ceased to be God's deacon. Were this not the case, we would be bound to state absolutism with no basis for resistance to tyranny of any and every kind* [emphasis added]. So, we are to obey God's ordinance to obey the civil authorities and fulfil our obligations until the state moves against God's ordinances. In all other cases we obey for the sake of our conscience and to avoid unnecessary punishment.[25]

The magistrate is to be a terror to those who practice evil and to be in praise of those who do good.[26] In our current world, mimicking all of history, that which is evil is frequently called good and that which is good is frequently called evil. The terms "evil" and "good" can only be defined by the Law of God (2 Timothy 3:16-17).

---

[25] Joe Boot, *Freedom, the Church and State Absolutism* (Ezra Institute, https://www.ezrainstitute.ca/resource-library/articles/freedom-the-church-and-state-absolutism/); July 15, 2020, accessed 8/23/2020.
[26] See Romans 13:3-4.

Likewise, the magistrate's authority to bear the sword against those who do evil must be within the parameters set forth by the *moral judicial Law of God*[27] and its general equity.[28, 29]

---

[27] Only those OT case laws (the "judicials") that have universal applications to all men in all places and all times are in view here as "moral" judicial laws. For example, rape, murder, theft, and kidnapping are sinful everywhere and are to be punished by the civil magistrate as a crime whether committed by a Hebrew, a Chinaman, a Peruvian, or an American. *Ceremonial* judicial laws (*along* with OT laws governing the Jews as a "body politick"), having expired with the ancient state of Israel in 70 AD at the hands of the Roman army and its brick by brick tearing down of the Temple (Matthew 24:1-2), are no longer in force except for any underlying moral principle(s) that may be contained within them. Laws of separation, for example, are still in force in the requirement that believers only marry in the Lord (1 Corinthians 7:39). Yet, a modern man may wear a cotton and polyester shirt (Deuteronomy 22:11). Other illustrations include laws forbidding sowing a field with different kinds of seeds (Deuteronomy 22:9;), specifics of crop rotation (Leviticus 25:3-7), dietary laws (Leviticus 11), concerns of Levirate marriage (Deuteronomy 25:5-10), cities of refuge (Numbers 35:6-34; Deuteronomy 4:41-43), laws of inheritance (Deuteronomy 21:15-17; Numbers 27:7-8), and the like.

[28] Defined literally as "universal justice" and is the application of the *general principles* of the Mosaic *moral* judicial laws (those with a basis or root in the 10 commandments) to modern situations and conditions (WCF 19.4*). By way of example, compare 1 Corinthians 9:8-14 and Deuteronomy 25:4. Here, the Apostle Paul applies the OT case law regarding the proper care and feeding of working livestock to the necessity of providing material (monetary and other) support to the ministers of God. If we are forbidden to "steal" from the ox by withholding grain while he threshes, how much more then that we do not steal from the minister as he labors for the benefit of the flock.

[29] A traditional application and illustration of general equity is the so-called parapet edict of Deuteronomy 22:8. This law required the construction of a rail or wall along the border perimeter of a flat roof to reduce the risk of a fall. In ancient Israel flat roofs were the norm and often used as places of family gathering and entertainment. The contemporary application of this ordinance is reflected in deck railings, highway guide rails, swimming pool fences and the like. And, as flat roofs with living and entertainment space are making a comeback, this precept has regained primary application!

For example, executing a person for petty shoplifting is forbidden. Civil sanctions decreed by the magistrate must follow the "punishment must fit the crime" paradigm (["eye for an eye" principle, *Lex Talionis*], Leviticus 24:17-23; Deuteronomy 19:21). Restitution for theft is required—not death or imprisonment (Exodus 22:1-4; Numbers 5:6-7; Leviticus 6:4; Luke 19:8).

In Romans 13:2, God forbids resisting the magistrate in two fundamental ways. First, we are *not* to be anarchists.[30] The Lord has given the civil magistrate to serve His purposes in the physical world until He returns on the Last Day. Until then, evil-doers require restraint so they not hinder God's redemptive purposes including the right of His created peoples to "a peaceful and quiet life" (1 Timothy 2:2). The civil magistrate is an example of a "common grace" institution.[31]

Second, we must obey the magistrate's *lawful* commands (this is true even if he is a non-Christian or worse, a tyrant[32]). He is always

---

[30] Anarchy is defined as opposition to the *institution* of very limited, Scripturally-restrained civil government (mini-archism) and is likewise forbidden in the family, church, and life of the individual. These governing domains are required to maintain strict allegiance to the Word of God and His moral Law.

[31] Controversies regarding the doctrine of "common grace" within the Reformed and Presbyterian communities notwithstanding, the author is strictly using the term to describe the non-salvific (thereby "common"), unmerited (hence "grace") providences of God to mankind irrespective of an individual's election or reprobation (e.g. rainfall, food, shelter, a good harvest, eminent gifts, good health, restraint of sin and crime). Arguably, a better term for this doctrine is "common Providence".

[32] Westminster Confession of Faith (WCF) 23.4.b.*

to be treated with honor and respect in a spirit of gentleness[33] ([LC] Q/A 127-128*). Nevertheless, these principles are not violated in the pointing out of significant sins and errors amongst inferiors, equals, and superiors (Galatians 6:1-5; Mark 6:18). All men are susceptible to being "called out" by the Law of God (Galatians 2:11-21).

As elucidated by the great Scottish Reformer John Knox,[34] the civil magistrate is intended to be, *first*, in covenant with God[35] (as he is God's servant) and, *second*, in pledge with the people and vowing to rule in accord with the precepts of God's law.[36] The people likewise are also to be in covenant with God and thereby in contract or covenant with the ruler to obey his *lawful* edicts.

These very important biblical principles were further expounded upon by Samuel Rutherford (a Scottish Presbyterian minister who ably served at the Westminster Assembly) in his classic work *Lex, Rex: The Law and the Prince*.[37, 38]

---

[33] This proves difficult for fallen mankind as we are often quick to mock our fallible superiors and to harshly criticize their errors. Nevertheless, all persons must battle against this sinful tendency.

[34] Richard L. Greaves, Theology and Revolution in the Scottish Reformation: Studies in the thought of John Knox (Christian University Press; 1st Printing Edition); 1980.

[35] 2 Kings 11:17.

[36] These principles may be, and often are, applied by way of humanly written state and Federal Constitutions. These documents *are* covenantal in nature having been ratified by the people (2 Kings 23:1-3). As such, they may be properly appealed to by Christians in disputes over civil law. The Apostle Paul did not hesitate to invoke his Roman citizenship as required for his defense (Acts 16:35-40, 22:25-28).

[37] Samuel Rutherford, *Lex, Rex: The Law and the Prince* (https://www.monergism.com/lex-rex-ebook); 1644, accessed 8/17/2020.

[38] The "Law is King"—as opposed to the "King is Law" (Divine Right of Kings).

Tyranny being a work of Satan, is not from God, because sin, either habitual or actual, is not from God: the power that is, must be from God; the magistrate, as magistrate, is good in nature of office, and the intrinsic end of his office, (Rom. xiii. 4) for he is the minister of God for thy good; and, therefore, a power ethical, politic, or moral, to oppress, is not from God, and is not a power, but a licentious deviation of a power; and is no more from God, but from sinful nature and the old serpent, than a license to sin. God in Christ giveth pardons of sin, but the Pope, not God, giveth dispensations to sin.[39]

When the magistrate breaks covenant in a high-handed and unrepentant fashion, he (or she)[40] may be resisted and removed from office and brought to justice by a variety of lawful means including, as an *absolute last resort*, the taking up of arms by the lesser magistrates.[41] These principles were explicitly applied in the second and fourth paragraphs of the 1776 colonial American *Declaration of Independence*.[42]

---

[39] Samuel Rutherford, *Lex, Rex*, p. 34.

[40] 2 Kings Chapter 11, particularly v. 20: "So all the people of the land rejoiced (cf. Proverbs 29:2), and the city was quiet after Athaliah had been put to death with the sword at the king's house."

[41] Matthew Trewhella, The Doctrine of the Lesser Magistrates: A Proper Resistance to Tyranny and a Repudiation of Unlimited Obedience to Civil Government (CreateSpace Independent Publishing Platform); 1st edition (2013).

[42] Britannica Online, *Declaration of Independence* (https://www.britannica.com/topic/Declaration-of-Independence/Text-of-the-Declaration-of-Independence), accessed 8/29/2020.

Note the following summary points regarding the biblical limitations of civil power.

- Crimes, *scripturally defined*, are those sins that are to receive punishment (sanctions) by the civil magistrate. Only here can true biblical justice and liberty be found. Alternatively, in the context of autonomous, humanistic "positive law," the citizenry will ultimately be subject to progressive tyranny. [43, 44]

- With a prophetic voice, the magistrate is to praise those who do good; alternatively, by way of proclaiming the fury of God's judicial wrath via Law, [45] he restrains/deters crime by making the people afraid (Deuteronomy 13:11; 17:33; 19:19b-20).

- Old Covenant Israel and her Law order are to be a model or standing template for the nations of the world (Deuteronomy 4:5-8). No New Testament Scriptures are found that negate or

---

[43] Defined by Herbert Schlossberg as an approach to law by which "the validity of the law (autonomously derived and independent of the moral Law of God [author's note, DO]) is dependent entirely on the fact of enactment; it does not have any force prior to that, nor may its validity be questioned after it is enacted by the constituted powers." *Idols for Destruction*, (Nashville: Thomas Nelson Publishers, 1983), p. 206. It is improper to contrast flawed legal positivity with natural law as it (NL) (as a *reliable* standard of moral righteousness) is marred by man's total depravity (Genesis 8:21). The SCOTUS Obergefell decision "legalizing" sodomite marriage demonstrates the folly of relying on natural law to provide true justice.

[44] Rousas John Rushdoony, *The Institutes of Biblical Law* (Phillipsburg, NJ. The Presbyterian and Reformed Publishing Company) 1973. pp. 101-106.

[45] On this earth and in eternity.

set aside this modeling (Matthew 5:17-20). Indeed, by the ultimate success of the Great Commission in the New Covenant era, the implications of the Deuteronomy text will be increasingly fulfilled[46] through all the earth—the nations, in time and great measure, will come to Christ and then rule by His Law (Isaiah 42:1-4; 10-13).

- The Great Commission (Matthew 28:18-20) commands the preaching of the Gospel to all the nations as the means by which the elect are saved and personally transformed and how then, as a result, the Kingdom of God and its sanctifying influence expands throughout the world affecting all areas and spheres of life.[47]

- Sections of WCF Chapters 20 and 23 repeatedly deploy the word "lawful." In WCF 23.2, the Confession refers to the "wholesome" laws of each commonwealth. Obviously, the "*Law*" mostly being referred to in this context is the moral Law of God. "*Wholesome laws*" can only refer to those civil man-made laws that are in *compliance* with the principles and general equity of

---

[46] An early covenantal fulfillment of this promise is seen in the proclamation of Artaxerxes (Ezra 7, most particularly verses 25-28).

[47] In the discipling of the nations via a program of extensive teaching regarding the moral Law of God and need for obedience to it. Obedience to the Law is **NEVER** to be used as a means of meriting salvation but **ONLY** as a guide to Godly sanctification.

the moral law of God. By way of example, pro-abortion statutes can in no way be considered "wholesome."

We must then ask—*have the civil magistrates acted biblically and therefore lawfully in their Covid-19 responses?* **No.**

Our Romans 13 text clearly and unequivocally gives the civil magistrate two *primary*[48, 49] duties: 1) be in praise to those who do good and 2) be a terror to those who do evil.

The second function includes defending the nation's borders[50] against invasion and the administration of a judicial system primarily in the adjudication of cases for those accused of capital crimes.

Non-capital crimes may be decided as well, provided they could not and were not successfully settled and administered person to person or in a family or informal civil court (neighbor to neighbor).

The magistrates may *not* interfere with ecclesiastical courts. A notable exception might be where a church court is acting in a manner

---

[48] Note that the state has not been given, as a *primary* duty, the protection of the health and "safety" of the citizenry. Any *secondary* role the state has in this arena is only related to limited and specific application of biblical ethics in the pursuit of justice (with justice only to be defined by God's Law).

[49] Rousas John Rushdoony, *The Institutes of Biblical Law*, pp. 58-62.

[50] This embraces also the application to a person(s) *voluntarily and legally* entering a nation from an area where a *serious* and highly *deadly* communicable disease is endemic so as to prevent general harm to the community and/or thwart evildoers who may wish to cause a nation detriment by way of communicable infectious agents.

that causes *it* to *trespass*[51] *into the magistrate's rightful sphere of authority* (which, biblically, is very limited). For example, if a church court would physically assault or torture its members[52] at large or perhaps take matters into its own hands by executing those proven guilty of biblical capital crimes without having been put to death by the state (as required by God's law). Scripturally, **only** the civil magistrate may bear the sword in the punishment of crime.

Given the preceding considerations, Scripture gives the magistrate, by way of general equity, a very limited *secondary* authority in the province of public health, namely isolation and quarantine.[53] As noted by Dr. Phillip G. Kayser,

> Lev. 13:45-46; Numb. 5:1-4; 12:14-16; 2 Kings 15:1-5 all deal with principles of quarantine. It is interesting however that it was not the state that had the power to determine a diseased or healed condition, but the priests (Lev. 13-14; Deut. 24:8). Furthermore, the priests did not have police power to investigate homes or to search for diseases that

---

[51] No governing domain may *ordinarily* trespass into the realm of another. The family has been given the "Rod of Correction", the magistrate, "the Sword" and the church, through her ordained officers, the "Keys to the Kingdom."

[52] The Court of High Commission, instituted in 1559. Wikipedia, "Court of High Commission" (https://en.wikipedia.org/wiki/Court_of_High_Commission); last edited on 17 August 2020, accessed 9/2/2020.

[53] Isolation refers to the separation of the contagious sick from all others except those necessarily involved in their spiritual and physical care. Quarantine refers to the temporary segregation (during the disease incubation period) of the physically well who were directly and meaningfully exposed to a serious, highly (not merely potentially) deadly communicable disease.

needed quarantining. Instead, citizens "brought" the infected person to the priest for examination (Lev. 13:2,9; 14:2). The need for citizen, church, and state to all be involved in the process helps to prevent abuses from occurring.[54]

It may be reasonably deduced that in modern nations, the work of the priest has been substantially replaced by the collective of the county health officer and his designates, families, and, where applicable, ecclesiastical authorities where applicable. In other words, while the OT passages referenced here were in the context of the Levitical priesthood and the ceremonial law, there are definitely moral (ethical) applications related to these considerations.[55]

Importantly, the individual suspected of having a communicable disease is required to be personally interviewed and examined. If the "patient" has no signs or symptoms or supporting diagnostic tests to suggest infection with a *serious*[56] contagious disease, then no isolation can be ordered. Likewise, only those in direct, non-incidental close contact with a person known definitively to have a highly communicable and dangerous infectious disease may be quarantined.

No direct civil penalty has been prescribed in Scripture for failure to obey the quarantine or isolation order, although a citizen could bring about a suit for damages or higher penalty *provided it was proven*

---

[54] Phillip G. Kayser, "Public Health and Limited Government" (https://kaysercommentary.com/Blogs/Public%20Health.md); 2015, accessed 8/15/2020.

[55] Deliberate attempts to spread one's own disease through unlawful contact.

[56] For example, small pox and plague but not measles, mumps, and rubella.

that sinful negligence of an isolation or quarantine order resulted in illness or death to another party.

While not impossible to demonstrate (see Typhoid Mary[57]), a successful conviction would be exceedingly difficult by God's rules of evidence (the case laws requiring two or three witnesses[58] which, we believe, *may* include in addition to eye-witnesses, circumstantial and forensic indicators). How does Tom prove that it was Mary's virus that infected him? And additionally, that she infected him with deliberation and premeditation?

Given the preceding discussion, it should be evident that arbitrary quarantine of the *multitude of a healthy and asymptomatic populace* by a central authority *without due process is absolutely unbiblical and unlawful* (centralization and consolidation of power is strongly frowned upon in God's Word, as it often leads to idolatry and tyranny [Genesis 11:1-9; 1 Samuel 8:6-18]).

Further, the Constitution of the State of Tennessee[59] (home state of the author) does not confer this authority to the governor.[60] Neither does the U.S. Constitution grant such authority to the Federal magistrate.

---

[57] Britannica Online, *Typhoid Mary* (https://www.britannica.com/biography/Typhoid-Mary), accessed 8/17/2020.

[58] Numbers 35:30; Deuteronomy 17:6-7, 19:15; Matthew 18:16; 2 Corinthians 13:1; 1 Timothy 5:19.

[59] *The Constitution of the State of Tennessee* (http://www.capitol.tn.gov/about/docs/TN-Constitution.pdf); Revised 2014, accessed 8/17/2020.

[60] Tennessee Constitution, Article 1 Sections 8 and 9.

In the Providence of God, our national and state constitutions and derived legal statutes were originally formulated (albeit quite imperfectly) upon the general principles of the Word of God. While the Apostle Paul did not enjoy such an environment, he did not hesitate to use Roman law (as a Roman citizen) to his advantage as circumstances dictated (see relevant texts in Acts).

Apart from the issue of unlawful quarantine, the law of God has been violated in a multitude of ways including those "wholesome" laws of the state of Tennessee[61] and the U.S. federal government.

To name but a few, lawful contracts have been disrupted.[62] Businesses were arbitrarily ordered closed.[63] Able-bodied, healthy men and women have been deprived of their right and duty before God to work and to take dominion over the earth.[64] As Paul has commanded, "If a man shall not work, he shall not eat" (2 Thessalonians 3:10). As nations are comprised of men, "a nation that shall not work shall not eat" is a very sobering indictment indeed.

"Executive orders" by Presidents and Governors, as heads of the executive branches in a republican form of government, have no

---

[61] Jeffery A. Cobble, Esquire, The Coronavirus Pandemic versus the Limits of Governmental Power (https://www.dropbox.com/s/llkfeso8qsp2tm7/The%20Coronavirus%20Pandemic%20vs.%20the%20Limits%20of%20Governmental%20Power.pdf?dl=0); April 2020, accessed 8/15/2020.

[62] Rent and mortgage obligations have been deferred by government fiat or simply ignored by the citizenry. Evictions and foreclosures too have been suspended also by fiat.

[63] A trespass against private property rights in violation of the 8th commandment ("thou shalt not steal").

[64] Genesis 1:28; 2:15; 2:19; 9:7.

lawful authority when directed towards the general citizenry as they possess no legislative capability. Law-making is solely the prerogative of the legislative branches of government.[65, 66]

To arbitrarily call men's various occupations and callings "essential" and "non-essential" is to demean and diminish that work. And, by forbidding the so called "non-essential" the opportunity to pursue their God-ordained tasks is to violate the ever important "equal protection under the law" principle[67] as prescribed by Scripture (Exodus 12:49).

The larger proportion of civil magistrates have, unlawfully to greater or lesser degrees (biblically and constitutionally), interfered with the public worship of Christ. Even if Covid-19 was the "plague of all plagues," *the civil magistrates cannot in any manner interfere with the ecclesiastical authority of the church, through her lawfully ordained officers, to decide as to what she should do in that circumstance.*

Christians have no duty or obligation to obey any of the magistrates' biblically lawless edicts (defined as any decree that would *clearly* cause a person to sin against God) as to do so would sinfully

---

[65] Tennessee State Constitution, Article 2 Section 3.

[66] U.S. Constitution, Article 1 Section 1.

[67] One law applicable to all men equally and without favoritism (see Proverbs 18:5; 22:2; 28:5; 29:6).

violate conscience[68] (WCF 20.2).[69] A proclamation issued lawlessly[70] by any superior (e.g. an executive order mandating that all citizens must wear a mask in public) that does not *necessarily* cause one to sin *may or may not be obeyed* depending on circumstances. Ordinarily, these diktats will be obeyed for wrath's sake.[71] At other times, and always with great wisdom and care, the order *may* be resisted in order to protect one's own sphere of authority from unlawful trespass.[72]

In summation, a multitude of actions by some federal, state, and local civil magistrates in response to the Coronavirus pandemic

---

[68] For an excellent summary of themes related to liberty of conscience, G. Brent Bradley, *Liberty of Conscience* (Westminster Presbyterian Church, Kingsport, TN, https://www.sermonaudio.com/sermoninfo.asp?m=t&s=814162054362); August 14, 2016, accessed 9/2/2020.

[69] WCF 20.2 "God alone is Lord of the conscience,[10] and hath left it free from the doctrines and commandments of men, which are, in anything, contrary to His Word; or beside it, if matters of faith, or worship.[11] So that, to believe such doctrines, or to obey such commands, out of conscience, is to betray true liberty of conscience:[12] and the requiring an implicit faith, and an absolute and blind obedience, is to destroy liberty of conscience, and reason also"[13] ([10] James 4:12; Rom. 14:4 [11] Acts 4:19, 5:29; 1 Cor. 7:23; Matt. 23:8–10; 2 Cor. 1:24; Matt. 15:9 [12] Col. 2:20,22–23; Gal. 1:10, 2:4–5, 5:1 [13] Rom. 10:17, 14:23; Isa. 8:20; Acts 17:11; John 4:22; Hosea 5:11; Rev. 13:12,16–17; Jer. 8:9).

[70] He is not in possession of the authority to issue any such decree.

[71] Obedience by the believer to "avoid trouble" as opposed to compliance rooted in a faulty notion that the Lord, by His law, requires such obedience. To place oneself under the rubric of the latter also violates the spirit of WCF 20.2.

[72] Examples of unlawful trespass include: unless otherwise delegated, a father may not permit outsiders to corporally discipline his children. Vigilantism is forbidden and represents citizen trespass into the magistrate's rightful realm of punishing criminals. Family-administered, at-home baptisms are to be rightly opposed by church officers.

are patently unlawful as they are unbiblical *and* in violation of the *wholesome* laws of the state(s).

In light of their lawlessness, civil magistrates may be legitimately impeached and removed from office by their respective state legislatures.[73] Those errant civil authorities who profess Christ should, unless they repent, face discipline by their churches. The Lord holds a very dim view towards those who break lawful oaths and vows (WCF Chapter 22).

Romans 13:2 is oft misunderstood as it is so frequently poorly exegeted. We see here that it is the very actions of the magistrates *themselves* during the Covid-19 pandemic debacle that illustrates what biblically-condemned resistance to lawful authority looks like.[74] Edicts were repeatedly issued for that which they possessed no legal authority to dispense.

The author has first-hand knowledge that a number of PCA congregations did not comply with civil edicts that they suspend public worship. And by doing so, these brothers and sisters are *guiltless* before the Lord.

The doctrine of the lesser magistrates declares,

---

[73] or by Congress for those federal officers who violate their oaths and vows in the issuance of lawless (unconstitutional) ordinances.

[74] An example unrelated to the present discussion but helpful in the illustration of the principle: the failure of the mayor of Portland, Oregon and the Governor of Oregon to order law enforcement to engage, arrest, and prosecute looters, violent protesters, and arsonists currently terrorizing the city on an almost daily basis.

that when the superior or higher civil authority makes an unjust/immoral law or decree, the lesser or lower ranking civil authority has both the right and duty to refuse obedience to that superior authority. If necessary, the lower authority may even actively resist the superior authority.[75]

It is important to note that a number of city-county district attorneys, sheriffs, and state troopers (Christian and non-Christian alike) stated they would not enforce unjust and unlawful pandemic-related edicts by their state and local superiors.

Rousas John Rushdoony notes the following in relation to "positive law" and public health:

> … if the law is positive in its function, **and if the health of the people is the highest law, then the state has total jurisdiction to compel the total health of the people.** The immediate consequence is a double penalty on the people. **First,** an omnicompetent state is posited, and a totalitarian state results. Everything becomes a part of the state's jurisdiction, because everything can potentially contribute to the health or the destruction of the people. **Because the law is unlimited, the state is unlimited. It becomes the business of the state, not to control evil, BUT TO CONTROL ALL MEN.** Basic to every totalitarian regime is a positive concept of the function of law [all caps added].

[75] Matthew Trewhella, The Doctrine of the Lesser Magistrates: A Proper Resistance to Tyranny and a Repudiation of Unlimited Obedience to Civil Government (CreateSpace Independent Publishing Platform); 1st edition (2013).

This means, **second**, that no area of liberty can exist for man; there is then no area of things indifferent, of actions, concerns, and thoughts which the state cannot govern in the name of public health. To credit the state with ability to minister to the general welfare, to govern for the general and total health of the people, is to assume an omnicompetent state, and to assume an all-competent state is to assume an incompetent people. **The state then becomes a nursemaid to a citizenry whose basic character is childish and immature.** The theory that law must have a positive function assumes thus that the people are essentially childish.[76]

Before moving to the second half of this chapter—the biblical limitations of *ecclesiastical* power—note the following nine summary points thus far regarding the biblical limitations of *civil* power.

1. Christ has explicitly declared his absolute authority[77] over all the created universe.[78] "All authority in heaven and on earth has been given to me." To oppose Christ here is to deny Him His Crown Rights over *all things* including the office (ministry) of civil government (magistracy) and its duties and limitations.

---

[76] Rousas John Rushdoony, *The Institutes of Biblical Law*, p. 102.

[77] Which is necessarily true as **He *is the Creator of all.***

[78] Matthew 28:18-20; Psalm 103:19.

2. The Bible provides for limited civil government with *TWO PRIMARY* duties: be in praise to those who do good and be a terror to those who act wickedly *and* criminally.

3. Biblically defined, the magistrate may only deal with evil as it relates to crimes.

4. The magistrate has *no primary* duty related to public health and safety. *The **CHIEF** responsibility for health and safety resides in and with the individual and family.*

5. Presidents and governors may issue executive orders but only with application to the functionaries of the executive offices and the agencies they oversee.

6. Executive orders issued to persons or agencies beyond the Executive branches of government are not legally binding on the citizenry and may be lawfully resisted.[79]

7. The mass quarantine of the healthy without due process is completely unlawful[80] and tyrannical.

8. Those magistrates who issued unlawful quarantine orders and other illicit edicts should be impeached and removed from office and be additionally subject to civil penalties (restitution for damages consequently inflicted).

---

[79] Phillip G. Kayser, *Problems with Executive Orders - A Preliminary Rant* (Kayser Commentary, https://kaysercommentary.com/Blogs/Executive%20Orders.md); 10/12/2015, accessed 8/25/2020.

[80] Unlawful biblically *and* by those "wholesome" laws of the various nations, states and commonwealths via their Constitutions.

9. Those magistrates who profess Christ and acted unlawfully similarly during the pandemic should be, upon failure to repent, subject to church discipline as they have violated their oaths and vows related to public office.

The Biblical Limitations of Ecclesiastical Power

EPHESIANS 1:22-23 (ESV): [22]*And he put all things under his feet and gave him as head over all things to the church,* [23]*which is his body, the fullness of him who fills all in all.*

The Bible and several chapters of the WCF teach unequivocally that the church is a separate and distinct organism from the state (and family) and thus exerts complete independence in its specific sphere of authority.[81, 82] Note how this authority is stated and biblically supported in the WCF (with Scripture proofs)[83]:

---

[81] Ecclesiastical matters alone, (WCF 31.4).

[82] As emphasized by Rev. Joseph Morecraft III, in his seminal 55-part sermon series, *History of the Reformation,* "The Church is not tax-exempt; the Church is non-taxable!" (Sermon Audio, https://www.sermonaudio.com/search.asp?currsection=sermonstopic&keyword=History+of+the+Reformation&keyworddesc=History+of+the+Reformation&seriesonly=true&sourceid=heritagerpchanove), accessed 8/25/2020.

[83] While the Scripture proofs in the WCF are generally printed in footnotes, they have been incorporated into the body of the text here for ease of reading.

WCF 25.1

The catholic or universal Church, which is invisible, consists of the whole number of the elect, that have been, are, or shall be gathered into one, **under Christ the Head thereof** [emphasis added]; and is the spouse, the body, the fullness of Him that filleth all in all (Ephesians 1:10, 22-23, 5:23,27,32; Colossians 1:18).

WCF 25.6

There is **no other head of the Church but the Lord Jesus Christ** [emphasis added] (Colossians 1:18; Ephesians 1:22). Nor can the Pope of Rome, in any sense, be head thereof (Matthew 23:8-10; 2 Thessalonians 2:3-4, 8-9; Revelation 13:6).

WCF 30.1

The Lord Jesus, **as King and Head of His Church**, hath therein appointed a government, in the hand of Church officers, **distinct** [emphases added] from the civil magistrate (Isaiah 9:6-7; Matthew 28:18-20; Acts 20:17-18; I Corinthians 12:28; I Thessalonians 5:12; I Timothy 5:17; Hebrews 13:7, 17, 24).

WCF 31.2

It belongeth to synods and councils, ministerially to determine controversies of faith, and cases of conscience; to set down rules and directions for the better ordering of the public worship of God, and **government of His Church** [emphasis added]; to receive complaints in cases of maladministration, and authoritatively to determine the same: which decrees and determinations, if consonant to the Word of God, are to be received with reverence and submission; not only for their agreement with the Word, but also for the power whereby they are made, as being an ordinance of God appointed thereunto in His Word (Matthew 18:17-20; Acts 15:15, 19, 24, 27-31; 16:4)

While it is a very weighty matter to challenge the directives of the civil magistrate, nevertheless, the decision to assemble or not assemble for public worship *rests solely* with the properly called and ordained elders of the church. Christ *ALONE* is the Lord of Conscience and is the *ONLY* Head of the Church. Neither the state, the CDC, the mayor, the public health department, WHO, nor "the people" by way of democracy, etc. has any authority whatsoever to interfere with her ecclesiastical decision-making.

The Elders, by way of *their* freedom of conscience in Christ, possess the Christian liberty and duty to do their *own biblical* analysis of any particular ecclesiastical situation (*in this case, the decision to engage in public worship despite edicts to the contrary from outsiders*), come to their *own* conclusions, and be free in their decision-making process from state interference.

It is hereby concluded that the biblical and Confessional data all irrefutably declare that the civil magistrate has no authority in the church regarding any ecclesiastical matter. As such, the civil magistrates may not, in any manner, interfere with the church's Covid-19 response.

Therefore, ***should the officers of Christ's Church have accepted the Covid-19 narrative a priori?*** **No.**

PROVERBS 18:17 (ESV): *The one who states his case first seems right, until the other comes and examines him.*

It must be explicitly stated that the overwhelming majority of church officers acted in good faith and with utmost sincerity, care, and concern during the early days of the pandemic.[84] While not unprecedented in history, Christ's Church has not—for many generations—been faced with the types of challenges brought about by the necessary conflation of medicine and theology as has been the case with Covid-19.

From the beginning, a multitude of conflicting opinions have and continue to flourish[85] regarding all facets of the Covid-19 narrative. Therefore, a Christian response to the Covid-19 pandemic

---

[84] Nevertheless, as all human action is to be examined in the light of Scripture, church officers and their conduct are not exempt from such scrutiny—especially when the response to the pandemic led to a suspension of the biblically-mandated gathering for public worship by the people of God.

[85] Often, these opinions, as framed, were/are outright contradictions. By the rules of logic (which are ethical in nature and from the hand of God) these incongruities violate the "Law of Non-Contradiction"—two contrasting things cannot, *simultaneously*, both be true. This observation alone should have led church leaders to proceed with extreme caution in their responses to the pandemic narrative.

presents a much more daunting and challenging task. But even these difficult circumstances can be reasonably sorted out by the careful use of the many tools the Lord has provided: *Scripture (as the ultimate and final authority), the Westminster Standards, biblical law, a proper presuppositional apologetic method, an exegetically sufficient understanding of biblical church-state relations, use of biblically wholesome man-made civil laws, and a Christian world and life view that self-consciously informs medical, scientific and statistical methodologies.*[86]

When the virus was initially making its way to the U.S. in early 2020, Dr. Fauci and most of the public health establishment were cautiously optimistic regarding Covid-19 outcomes in the United States. Dr. Fauci recognized that "the denominator" (total number of Covid-19 infected patients irrespective of symptoms status) was likely "high." He stated in a February *NEJM* editorial (online edition):

"If one assumes that the number of asymptomatic or minimally symptomatic cases is several times as high as the number of reported cases, the case fatality rate may be considerably less than 1%. *This suggests that the overall clinical consequences of Covid-19 may ultimately be more akin to those of a severe seasonal influenza (which has a case fatality rate of approximately 0.1%)* or a pandemic influenza (similar to those

---

[86] In addition, it is very important to add here the necessity of a proper biblical anthropology. Natural man is thoroughly sinful, totally depraved, and capable of all sorts of evil (Genesis 6:5; Romans 3:10-18; Jeremiah 17:9-10; Mark 7:21-23).

in 1957 and 1968) **rather than** a disease similar to SARS or MERS, which have had case fatality rates of 9 to 10% and 36%, respectively [all emphases added]."[87]

When "cases"[88] began to increase (primarily attributable to exponentially greater numbers being tested—many of whom were asymptomatic), the media and public health presentations became increasingly hysterical, fearful, and panic-laden. Citing the now discredited IHME[89] and Imperial College, London computer modeling,[90] they shouted, "Plague! Plague!" Many thousands of puzzled physicians, virologists, epidemiologists, and intrigued lay persons around the globe looked outside and saw no plague. Except for a tiny number of "hot spots," *directly*[91] attributable deaths and hospitalizations were

---

[87] Anthony Fauci et al. *Covid-19 — Navigating the Uncharted* (New England Journal of Medicine; February 28, 2020; online at https://www.nejm.org/doi/full/10.1056/NEJMe2002387), accessed 8/22/2020.

[88] The term "case(s)" has been subtly redefined by the press and public health officials to mean any person with a "positive" Covid-19 test—even though the patient may not be proven infected or was/is symptomless.

[89] Institute for Health Metrics and Evaluation.

[90] Which predicted 2 million or more deaths in the United States and at least 500,000 in the United Kingdom. Obviously, these "prophecies" were wrong by orders of magnitude.

[91] Dying *FROM* Covid-19 and not merely *"WITH"* it (a positive RT-PCR test in the absence of Covid-19 signs and symptoms that *alone* explain the patient's condition and resultant death). For example, an elderly, chronically ill man with obesity, hypertension, oxygen-dependent COPD, severe chronic kidney disease, and heart failure presents with pneumonia and respiratory failure requiring a respirator. Pneumococcus bacteria are isolated from his lung tissues and blood. A nasal swab RT-PCR test is done and is "positive" for Covid-19. The patient dies and is (and certainly will be) labeled a Covid-19 death despite the fact

observed to be quite low. No matter. The "Plague!" mantra was repeated over and over again.

Alas, here we are in late August 2020 and a plague, as historically described, remains unseen. Nevertheless, the public is subject to relentless[92] propaganda: the necessity of a vaccine as *"the only way out of this"*; mask mandates (or euphemistically, "face coverings") as the *best* means to prevent the spread of Covid-19[93]; and other draconian physical distancing measures that were originally deemed temporary to "flatten the curve" but now seemingly have no end.

In the suspension of corporate worship, the larger body of global, "conservative and evangelical" Protestant Christianity revealed (at least in part) a subconscious abandonment of the foundational components of biblical apologetics: the necessity of understanding the world around us by way of a vigorous and thoroughgoing *Christian world view analysis*.

---

he expired from bacterial pneumonia and sepsis in the setting of a multitude of serious medical co-morbidities.

[92] Literally, a form of psychological terrorism which includes 24/7 presentations of death counts and "cases" as well as the conspicuous absence of any "good news" regarding the pandemic.

[93] Despite 100 years of investigation, the efficacy of public face masking in the prevention of viral respiratory disease has never been conclusively shown to confer any meaningful benefit. In the early days of the pandemic, CDC and WHO, citing these past studies, discouraged the use of masks. Suddenly, naming "new" research, they have turned on a dime. That these studies are mostly poorly designed observational and computer modeling constructs has been ignored along with the fact that overturning 100 years of data cannot be reliably done by new research in the span of a few months. Dr. Yeager addresses this further in chapter 5.

To momentarily review some basic concepts of worldview analysis, it is best to start here: there are no *raw* facts—only *interpreted* facts. As such, all men interpret all raw facts *through the lens* of their worldview (aka their *religion*)—*ALWAYS. All men, self-consciously or not, are religious as someone or something is transcendently the focus of their attentions and affections and forms the basis for their views on "how the world works" and "what's the meaning of life."* Hence, there is no neutrality amongst mankind's various worldviews.[94] Each person's worldview is shaped and framed solely by the Word of God (*sola* and *tota Scriptura*) or it's not. It's either Christ or the world. There are no alternatives. The principle of "non-neutrality" is to be consistently applied to all of life including our various scientific endeavors *and* in the interpretation of scientific data.

The doctrine of non-neutrality in concert with the Great Commission, a proper exegesis of Romans 13, and the principles of the Dominion (Creation) Mandate[95] instructs us that civil magistrates, in their capacity as civil magistrates, are accountable to God and His Law for their actions.

While many of the people at WHO, CDC, local and state public health departments, etc. are mostly able and intelligent individuals with good intentions and true expertise with regards to certain technical facets of coronavirus analysis, they nonetheless swim in their own worldview and *will interpret* Covid-19 with that worldview. And they will *NOT* be neutral in that interpretation.

---

[94] Or religions; see Matthew 12:30.
[95] Genesis Chapter 1-2, 8-9.

Christians must keep in mind that the majority of public health and other government officials currently guiding their populaces (and actually terrorizing them in many jurisdictions) regarding the coronavirus pandemic are immersed in the dominant worldview of our culture: atheistic materialism (AM).

AM is totally antithetical to a biblical Christian worldview and has foisted its values upon what is now the former "Christian West" or "Christendom" (*all the while aided and abetted by an apathetic church whose love has grown increasingly cold in love of the Law of God as it pertains to personal and societal sanctification*). Some examples of this include a demand for public acceptance and *affirmation* of homosexualism and other grotesque sexual perversions, abortion, infanticide, eugenics, transgenderism, transhumanism, Darwinianism, racism, massive indebtedness, "lawful" counterfeiting of currency and calling it "QE or fiscal stimulus," *unequal* protection under judicial law , false weights and measures, lying, falsification of data, hatred of the biblical family structure, socialism, unjust taxation, and on and on and on.

AM hates the Law of God, and yet its adherents are irrationally in constant agitation with the world around them over what they view as "moral and just." It is devastatingly "Messianic" in character and therefore in total *defiance* of the First Commandment of our Lord.[96]

In light of the foregoing, Christians should *necessarily assume* that those adhering to this worldview or some facet of it are ordinarily,

---

[96] And consequently, its adherents strenuously engage in "total warfare" against God's people.

and unless proven otherwise,[97] **blind guides** in the many areas of life to which they speak. They are the "blind leading the blind."

Failed public health prophecies[98] of the relatively recent past provide confirmation: HIV-AIDS, bird (avian) flu, swine flu x 2, Zika virus, anthrax, E. Coli, West Nile Virus, SARS-CoV-1, MERS, Ebola and Mad Cow disease to name but a few.

Having said this, we can take comfort in the knowledge that (a) because of God's "common Providence" and (b) because "the works of the law" are written on the hearts of all men, the unregenerate will (despite their total depravity) borrow heavily from the Christian world and life view in an attempt to understand the world in which they live. As such, they will more or less "get right" many things in this world.

Nonetheless, errors of epic proportion are unavoidable, too. Citizens of the U.S. are seeing this scenario play out right now before our very eyes in the disastrous magisterial, ecclesiastical, and cultural responses to the Covid-19 pandemic.[99]

It may be objected that the Bible has nothing to say about coronavirus. This is true. But the Bible has much to say about how we can *ethically* interpret and apply the science of coronavirus. (The

---

[97] By thorough analysis of whatever topic is at hand in the light of the *principles* (general equity) set forth in the entire Word of God.

[98] The establishment media, as mouthpieces for the public health ruling classes, predicted with urgency that these diseases would result in much morbidity and, very likely, high levels of mortality. Given a "prophetic" batting average of .000, it is reasonably concluded that the purpose of these narratives was not a genuine concern with medical accuracy but to repeatedly condition, stoke, and foment fear amongst the populace.

[99] See Dr. Yeager's important discussion in Chapter 5.

science, in and of itself, is technical in nature and is not ethical, but the conduct of scientific endeavors and its interpretation and application most certainly are principled and thereby subject to scrutiny by the Law of God).

The CDC/WHO/Mainstream Media Portrayal of Covid-19 Is Not True

Elsewhere in this volume, Dr. Joel Yeager ably explores the particulars as to the multitude of ways by which the Covid-19 narrative has turned the traditional medical and common-sense approach to viral respiratory disease on its head.[100] Here, the author will review several salient data points demonstrating the *complete absence of a medical basis* for the draconian world-wide lockdowns which triggered the widespread shuttering of churches for public worship and are hence relevant to our discussion.

Huge swaths of the general population have accepted the media portrayal of this disease even though *their own observations and experiences explicitly deny it.* This has resulted in a multitude of decidedly

---

[100] See also, Daniel O'Roark, *A Brief Covid-19 Analysis and Its Implications for the Church, Part One* (Aquilla Report, https://www.theaquilareport.com/a-brief-covid-19-analysis-and-its-implications-for-the-church/); March 30, 2020, accessed 8/29/2020; and Daniel O'Roark, *A Brief Covid-19 Analysis and Its Implications for the Church, Part Two* (Aquilla Report, https://www.theaquilareport.com/a-brief-covid-19-analysis-and-its-implications-for-the-church-part-2/); April 30, 2020, accessed 8/29/2020.

adverse consequences.[101] In a previous essay, the author stated the following:

> The potentially disastrous situation we find ourselves in has come about, in part, by a totally inexplicable desire by our magistrates and public health officials to portray Covid-19 as a monstrous, highly contagious and virulent virus by which one places their life at risk just by being around [even casually] an infected person. That this is balderdash is proven by the "eyeball test" alone.[102]

Where are the endless streams of "body" trucks, overflowing morgues, mass graves everywhere, and the eminently and easily measurable large increases in all-cause mortality? These were and are nowhere to be found. Only a minority of the general population even personally knows anyone who has tested "positive" for SARS-Cov-2 let alone succumbed either *from or with* Covid-19.

To begin with, it is important to understand that there are many problems with Covid-19 testing. The primary test being used to "diagnose" SARS-Cov-2 infection is the reverse transcriptase polymerase chain reaction (RT-PCR). It is a nucleic acid amplification test: it looks for viral nucleic acid gene sequences (in this case, messenger RNA) in a particular tissue sample and then amplifies them through repeated test cycles. Importantly, test accuracy weakens

---

[101] Spiritually, medically, politically, economically, and psychologically.

[102] Daniel O'Roark, *A Brief Covid-19 Analysis and Its Implications for the Church, Part Two.*

greatly as the number of amplification cycles needed to "see" the viral genes sequences increases.

Given the extremely small nature of these particles when looked for in nasopharyngeal specimens (and other samples from the lungs and bronchial tree), it is essentially a "looking-for-a-needle-in-a-haystack" type of test given the huge number of companion microbes present at any point in time in the human respiratory tract.

Secondary testing includes acute and convalescent sera (blood plasma) which check for the presence of antibodies presumptively indicative of acute infection (IgM antibodies) or past exposure but not currently infected (IgG antibodies). The very large numbers of reported "positive tests" are including *BOTH* positive IgG and RT-PCR results.[103] Obviously, this dubious tactic has greatly inflated the number of "Covid cases".

Additionally, the RT-PCR test, contrary to popular belief, *does not prove the presence and number*[104] of actively replicating viral particles but *only* reflects the detection of a snippet of messenger RNA gene sequences thought compatible with SARS-Cov-2. In essence, the RT-PCR is a "viral body parts" test. The presence of these gene

---

[103] CNN Wire, CDC and 11 states acknowledge mixing results of viral and antibody tests (https://fox4kc.com/tracking-coronavirus/cdc-and-11-states-acknowledge-mixing-results-of-viral-and-antibody-tests/); May 23, 2020., accessed 9/8/2020. In other words, if a patient initially tests positive with a nasal swab and then later has a positive serum antibody test, that same patient is counted twice in the Covid tally.

[104] It is true that positive results with few test cycles *implies* the presence of a large number of viral particles. But, most importantly, the presence of large numbers of actively replicating viral particles will be seen in *SICK* people, not asymptomatic persons.

sequences (in whole or in part) *does not* necessarily mean that the detected nucleic acid fragments[105] represent an *intact, potentially infectious* virion.[106] It could be a virion already "dead" by the actions of the host's immune system. It could be a "passenger" virion merely present in the nasopharynx but not causing disease.[107] It could very possibly be positive from cross-reactivity with one of the four "common" corona virus strains. Or it could even be RNA from other sources including the body's own cells via cellular exosome extrusion.[108]

An essay by Torsten Engelbrecht and Konstantin Demeter[109] amplifies the highly problematic nature of RT-PCR testing (which includes the absence of a true "gold standard")[110] in the diagnosis of

---

[105] the gene sequences present in nasopharyngeal secretions and collected via swab techniques.

[106] Defined by Oxford Dictionary as, "the complete, infective form of a virus outside a host cell, with a core of RNA or DNA and a capsid."

[107] It is estimated that the human body contains 1-4 trillion cells, **and, at any given time, 100 trillion viruses are present on or within the body.** Despite this, humans are almost "never" sick (germ theory versus terrain theory debate).

[108] Zhang Wei, Zhang Bing, et al *Expression of miRNAs in plasma exosomes derived from patients with atrial fibrillation* (Clinical Cardiology, (https://onlinelibrary.wiley.com/doi/full/10.1002/clc.23461?campaign=wolearlyview), September 17, 2020, accessed 10/5/2020.

[109] *Covid-19 PCR Tests are Scientifically Meaningless* (Off Guardian, https://off-guardian.org/2020/06/27/covid19-pcr-tests-are-scientifically-meaningless/); June 27, 2020, accessed 8/29/2020.

[110] A "gold standard test" is the best available diagnostic test for determining whether a patient does or does not have a disease or condition. For example, if one were testing the accuracy of various pregnancy tests, the pregnancy itself is the "gold standard."

SARS-Cov-2 which is manifested by the Covid-19 syndrome (a clinical collection of signs and symptoms).

At the end of the day, there are essentially *three* coronavirus outcomes one needs to care about: death, severe disease that does not cause demise but requires an ICU stay +/- respirator support, and non-ICU hospitalization rates. *The number of people in a region with a positive test (so called "cases") does not matter at all as long as the aforementioned adverse outcomes occur at a very low rate.* By all current accounts and evidence, these rates are indeed very low and have been since the beginning of the Covid-19 fiasco.[111]

Next, it is extremely important to briefly review the principles of Bayesian statistical analysis[112] and its role in the proper interpretation of medical test results. These principles have been largely "thrown out the window" in the Covid-19 paradigm. In the minds of many, a "positive" Covid-19 test means one "has" Covid-19. As will be demonstrated, this is patently false as this assumes a test specificity[113] of 100% (which is virtually never true of any diagnostic test).

---

[111] A small number of true "Covid hotspots" excluded. A "true" Covid-19 hotspot is a place where many are seriously ill with the disease and is not simply declared present because of a large number of positive test results alone and divorced from the clinical context.

[112] Bayesian statistical analysis and its "Bayes Theorem" is frequently used in the field of medicine and its use widely accepted.

[113] Test *specificity* refers to the number of persons with a positive test result who actually have the disease in question. A test with 100% specificity represents a test with no false positives. Test *sensitivity* refers to the percentage of patients *WITH* the disease in question who will test positive for that disease. It measures the ability of a test to detect a disease. A test with, for example, a sensitivity of 30% will miss the disease when it is present 70% of the time. Such a test is essentially worthless from a diagnostic capability standpoint. An assay

The larger body of the medical establishment *believes* that the RT-PCR for SARS-Cov-2 has a specificity of 97-98% which translates into a 2-3% *false positive*[114] rate.

To put sensitivity and specificity in a proper diagnostic perspective, one must know the *prevalence or pre-test probability of disease* in the population to which the test will be applied. For example, 16-year-old girls with sharp stabs of chest pain almost never have coronary artery disease; hence, a positive exercise treadmill test in that setting almost always represents a "false positive" study. The post-test probability of coronary disease remains quite low despite the abnormal result.

Using data obtained from the Tennessee Department of Health[115] obtained prior to April 18, 2020,[116, 117] one is able to reasonably elucidate the prevalence of a "positive" Covid-19 RT-PCR test in a population of people with flu-like symptoms. In the context of these strict and well-defined prerequisites for testing, the number of symptomatic Tennesseans "testing positive" for Covid-19 was about 8%. Therefore, ***assuming*** a 70% test sensitivity (or 30% false negative

---

with 100% sensitivity and 100% specificity (almost never present in the "real world") will identify all patients who have the disease and exclude all patients who do not have it.

[114] Meaning the test is positive but the patient does not have the targeted disease.

[115] Tennessee Department of Health (https://www.tn.gov/health/cedep/ncov.html), accessed 8/29/2020.

[116] After this date, virtually anyone who wanted a test could get one regardless of whether flu-like symptoms were present or not.

[117] Prior to April 18th, to be tested, the patient had to have symptoms ("flu-like illness") suggesting infection with SARS-Cov-2 *and* a negative *influenza* screen.

rate) and a hypothetical test specificity of 100% (0% false positive rate), the prevalence or pre-test probability of a "positive" Covid-19 PCR test in symptomatic Tennesseans is about 11%.

Utilizing a University of Illinois, Chicago calculator developed by Professor Alan Schwartz[118] with an assumed symptomatic disease prevalence of 11%, RT-PCR sensitivity of 70%,[119] specificity of 98%, and 600,000 people tested,[120] the post-test probability of SARS-Cov-2 infection in *symptomatic* Tennesseans is about 82%. This would mean that amongst those with a positive test, 18% *did not* have the disease and the results are therefore appropriately labeled "false positive".

When testing became very widespread (see footnote #115), *large numbers of people with no symptoms or minimal symptoms* (runny nose but not necessarily with typical flu-like symptoms such as fever, cough, muscle aches, shortness of breath) presented for testing. Suddenly, numbers became almost meaningless. Why? Because the prevalence of disease is always lower in asymptomatic populations. Exactly how low in relation to Covid-19 is unknown, again due to the lack of a robust gold standard test.[121] If a disease prevalence of 1% is assumed

---

[118] University of Illinois, Chicago, *Professor Alan Schwartz Web Server* (http://araw.mede.uic.edu/cgi-bin/testcalc.pl), accessed 8/29/2020.

[119] This number has been assumed by CDC and other public health officials. For the purposes herein, it is assumed to be true but the lack of a gold standard test for SARS-CoV-2 is highly problematic.

[120] Estimated number of tests performed in Tennessee as of April 18, 2020.

[121] Some may object that viral cultures for SARS-CoV-2 have been performed and this is true. The question here is one of reliability. To date, there is no evidence that the isolated

in an asymptomatic or minimally symptomatic population, the post-test probability of disease is a paltry 28%. Stated another way, **82% of those with a positive test *DO NOT* have the disease.**

As can be seen, the intense CDC-WHO push for "testing-testing-testing" of all-comers has led to very misleading results. Given the long-held and time-tested Bayesian probability principles, this can only reflect one or both of two things: 1) *massive incompetence or* 2) *a deliberate misrepresentation of the* truth and a violation of the 9th commandment, "Thou Shall Not Bear False Witness."

This explains the large spike in positive test results with an "all comers" testing paradigm during the 2020 summer months and is responsible for the hysterical media presentation of increasingly larger numbers of daily Covid-19 "cases" and a "massive second wave." Never before have health care providers routinely tested asymptomatic or minimally symptomatic persons for acute viral respiratory illness of various etiologies—most especially during the summer months. The poor positive predictive value of a "positive" test explains why.

Finally, before moving on to the next section, we take a brief but necessary excursus regarding the unprecedented bastardization of vital statistics by the CDC when it comes to reporting and tallying Covid-19 deaths.

SARS-CoV-2 virus has been successfully purified/filtered. In keeping with Koch's and Rivers postulates, purification (by implication in their writings) is vital so as to verify that the virus in question is a unique and actually causing the disease syndrome and not some other pathogen, viral or non-viral.

In a move that defies belief, CDC instructed physicians early on during the lockdowns to list Covid-19 as the primary cause of death on death certificates, even ***WHEN IT IS ONLY SUSPECTED WITH NO TESTING REQUIRED:***

> Covid-19 should be reported on the death certificate for all decedents where the disease caused ***or is assumed to have caused or contributed to death*** [emphasis in original]. Certifiers should include as much detail as possible based on their knowledge of the case, medical records, laboratory testing, etc. If the decedent had other chronic conditions such as COPD or asthma that may have also contributed, these conditions can be reported in Part II. (See attached Guidance for Certifying COVID-19 Deaths).[122]

Exact cause of death determinations done in good faith have always been difficult to do with precision. Here, physicians are being explicitly instructed to forgo meticulousness in what seems to be a deliberate attempt to drive up the number of reported Covid-19 fatalities. Additionally, as noted by H. Ealy, M. McEvoy, et. al.,

> Had the CDC used its industry standard, *Medical Examiners' and Coroners' Handbook on Death Registration and Fetal*

---

[122] Steven Schwartz, PhD, COVID-19 Alert No. 2: New ICD code introduced for COVID-19 deaths
(Centers for Disease Control, https://www.cdc.gov/nchs/data/nvss/coronavirus/Alert-2-New-ICD-code-introduced-for-COVID-19-deaths.pdf); March 24, 2020, accessed 8/30/2020.

Death Reporting Revision 2003, as it has for all other causes of death for the last 17 years, the COVID-19 fatality count would be approximately 90.2% lower than it currently is.[123]

These actions are, of course, grossly immoral and unjust given how these data have driven and will continue to drive incredibly important public health policy decisions.

While overall Covid-19 mortality slightly exceeds that of influenza, understanding these data in a proper context requires exploration of death rates in various age groups. It is now known that almost 50% of Covid-19 related deaths occur in the extreme elderly—most of whom also have multiple, serious medical co-morbidities and often reside in nursing homes or other long-term care facilities.

It is also generally accepted by the CDC and WHO that the percentage of people (across all age groups) who die with/from SARS-CoV-2 infection[124] is about 0.2%. For people younger than 45, the infection fatality rate is almost 0%. For 45 to 70, it is probably about 0.05-0.3%.[125] For influenza, the infection fatality rate is about 0.1%.

[123] H. Ealy, M. McEvoy, et. al., *If COVID Fatalities Were 90.2% Lower, How Would You Feel About Schools Reopening?* (Children's Health Defense, https://childrenshealthdefense.org/news/if-covid-fatalities-were-90-2-lower-how-would-you-feel-about-schools-reopening/); July 24, 2020, accessed 9/15/2020.

[124] That infection being with or without symptoms (the latter never symptomatic group identified via antibody testing).

[125] Patricia Claus, *Up to 300 Million People May Be Infected by Covid-19, Stanford Guru John Ioannidis Says* (Greek Reporter, https://usa.greekreporter.com/2020/06/27/up-to-300-million-people-may-be-infected-by-covid-19-stanford-guru-john-ioannidis-says/); June 27, 2020, accessed 9/9/2020.

Sweden, which largely avoided draconian lock-down measures (and was roundly criticized as its approach was predicted to "certainly lead to unprecedented deaths"), has in reality experienced "middle-of-the-pack" mortality statistics when compared to other nations and various American states and commonwealths (some imposing very strict self-quarantine measures).

In meticulous work by David Stockman, it is irrefutably shown that most Swedish coronavirus deaths occurred in extremely aged, chronically ill individuals who were already approaching the end of life. These patients, irrespective of any contracted viral respiratory infection, may be reasonably anticipated to have a life expectancy of less than one year given their extreme frailty and pre-existing disease states. Per Stockman,

Number of WITH-Covid deaths/ Population/Rate per 100,000 by age cohort:

➢ 0-9 years: 1/1.22 million/ *0.08* per 100,000;
➢ 10-19 years: 0/1.19 million/ *0.0* per 100,000;
➢ 20-29: 10/1.31 million/ *0.77* per 100,000;
➢ 30-39 years: 16/1.37 million/ *1.16* per 100,000;
➢ 40-49 years: 45/1.31 million/ *3.42* per 100,000;
➢ 50-59 years: 162/1.27 million/ *12.8* per 100,000;
➢ 60-69 years: 398/1.14 million/ *34.8* per 100,000;
➢ 70-79 years: 1,250/.917 million/ *128.7* per 100,000;
➢ 80-90 years: 2,408/.425 million/ *567.0* per 100,000;

> 90 years plus: 1,512/.119 million/ *1,271.0* per 100,000.[126]

A close examination of these data provides irrefutable confirmation that in persons under age 60, Covid-19 related deaths occur at an extraordinarily low rate and are fewer in number than those seen typically (in the United States) from influenza/pneumonia across all age groups.[127]

In an earlier essay, Stockman demonstrated similar findings in U.S. populations, pointing out that the degree of lockdown had no correlation to outcomes:

… But there is zero correlation:

> *California*: Heavy lockdown, *4.6* deaths per 100,000;
> *Iowa*: No lockdown, *4.3* deaths per 100,000;
> *Texas*: Light lockdown, *2.4* deaths per 100,000;
> *Washington state*: Heavy lockdown, *10.0* deaths per 100,000;
> *Colorado*: Inconsistent lockdown, *12.2* deaths per 100,000;
> *Georgia*: Late Lockdown now lifted, *10.0* deaths per 100,000;

---

[126] David Stockman, *The Tyranny of Group Think* (Lew Rockwell.com, https://www.lewrockwell.com/2020/08/david-stockman-the-tyranny-of-groupthink/); August 22, 2020, accessed 8/29/2020.

[127] CDC, *Influenza/Pneumonia Mortality by State* (https://www.cdc.gov/nchs/pressroom/sosmap/flu_pneumonia_mortality/flu_pneumonia.htm); 2018, accessed 9/8/2020.

- *Maine*: Heavy Lockdown, *3.8* deaths per 100,000;
- *Massachusetts*: Heavy Lockdown, *45.7* deaths per 100,000...

... Indeed, with each passing update, the CDC data itself becomes an ever more dispositive indictment of the madness the Donald's doctors have imposed on the nation. It is now strikingly clear, in fact, that when it comes to Covid-19 there are three nations in America, and *that the attempt to shoe-horn them into a one-size fits all regime of state control is tantamount to insane* [emphasis added].

There is first the *Kids Nation* of some 61 million persons under 15 years, where even by the CDCs elastic definitions there have been just 5 *WITH* Covid deaths thru April 28. You needn't even bother with the zero-ridden fraction of 1 per 100,000 (its actually 0.008) to make the point.

That is to say, last year there were about 44,000 deaths among the Kids Nation – so coronavirus accounts for just 0.011% of the total, and in no sane world would it be a reason for shutting down the schools.

Of course, the Virus Patrol insists that the school closures are an unfortunate necessity because otherwise the Kids Nation would take the virus home to the *Parents/Workers Nation*. That is the 215 million citizens between 15 and 64, *who account for the overwhelming share of commerce, jobhold-ers and GDP* [emphasis added].

Yet according to the CDC, there have been just 8,267 deaths *WITH* Covid in this massive expanse of the population, which figure represents a mortality rate of, well, 3.6 per 100,000.

But here's the thing. The normal total mortality rate for the 15-64 years old population is 335 per 100,000. So, we are talking about shutting down the entire economy owing to a death rate to date which amounts to 1.1% of normal mortality in the *Parents/Workers Nation.*

Finally, we have ***Grandparents/Great Grandparents Nation,*** comprised of 52 million citizens. But they account for 32,000 or nearly 80% of the *WITH* Covid deaths as of April 28 – with 15,000 of these being among those 85 years and older.

By way of computation, that's 61 deaths per 100,000 for the group as a whole and 230 per 100,000 for the 85 years and older.

Stated differently, the risk of death posed by Covid-19 is ***7,600X greater for Grandparents/Great Grandparents Nation overall than for Kids Nation, and 29,000 times greater for the several million Great-Grandparents*** afflicted with severe comorbidity and likely as not to be in the care of a nursing home [emphasis added].

Needless to say, it did not take a catastrophic experiment with Lockdown Nation to figure this out. It was already known from China and the history of other coronaviruses [emphasis added].[128]

The "Devilish" Doctrine of the Asymptomatic Covid-19 "Super-Spreader"[129]

Make no mistake about it. The oft stated and highly touted thesis that asymptomatic spread from the "apparently" well is *the* primary source of Covid-19 disease transmission *has absolutely not been proven*. And yet it was and still remains the *foundational* presupposition of the near global societal lock-down measures and the pandemic narrative itself. Never before in human history have asymptomatic persons with no known exposure to a contagious illness been subject to widespread home quarantine demands—and all of this without due process.

---

[128] David Stockman, *The Three Nations of Covid and a Windbag Named Fauci* (Lew Rockwell.com, https://www.lewrockwell.com/2020/05/david-stockman/the-three-nations-of-covid-and-a-windbag-named-fauci/) May 2, 2020, accessed 8/29/2020. See also footnote #37 in chapter 2.

[129] This concept is also addressed as myth #2 in chapter 2.

In light of this faux foundational premise, it was posited that the only way to "stop" the pandemic was to place gargantuan swaths of the populace under what was effectively "house-arrest."

Historically, only the already sick or those at high risk for *complicated* illness were isolated. Meaningfully exposed patients were briefly quarantined, and only then if the disease in question was highly contagious and notably deadly, such as smallpox. Even with the much-feared smallpox, the whole populace was not isolated or quarantined.

In Chapter 2, Dr. Joel Yeager deals more comprehensively with the medical refutation of other medical "myths" endemic to the Covid-19 narrative. The author here adds his own brief medical analysis summarizing what he believes to be a most ***CRUCIAL OBSERVATION***:

If the notion that asymptomatic persons are the primary sources of viral respiratory disease transmission is widely accepted as true, then arbitrary and unlimited intrusions by the state will become normative, with the end result being unyielding medical and societal tyranny.

In the author's view (and parroting Rushdoony), this paradigm represents an EXISTENTIAL THREAT to Christian and societal liberty and must be vigorously opposed.

It is true that asymptomatic humans infected by a communicable respiratory disease can potentially (albeit rarely) spread that disease while having no symptoms. This is especially factual of measles but much less so for most other viral etiologies of acute respiratory illness. Studies of influenza viruses have revealed that infectivity is related to the degree of viral shedding which in turn tightly corresponds to clinical severity (high fever, etc.).[130] *Sick people shed a logarithmically higher volume of virus than asymptomatic persons during coughing and/or sneezing. "The sicker you are the more virus you will shed."*[131]

Viruses can only replicate (reproduce) inside the cells of a host organism (be it human, other mammal, bird, bacteria, etc.). During the replication process host cells are killed proportional to the magnitude of reproduction and it is the body's immune and inflammatory responses to cellular death that leads to clinical signs and symptoms (fever, chills, body aches, coughing, sneezing, etc.) of illness. The magnitude of cellular death is generally proportional to the degree of symptoms.

---

[130] Eleni Patrozou, MD Leonard Mermel, DO, Does Influenza Transmission Occur from Asymptomatic Infection or Prior to Symptom Onset? (Public Health Reports, https://www.dropbox.com/s/19nvb1y04c0o4w0/Does%20Influenza%20Transmission%20Occur%20from%20Asymptomatic%20Infection_Patrozou%20and%20Mermel.pdf?dl=0); March-April 2009, Volume 124, accessed 8/31/2020.

[131] Lincoln L. H. Lau, Benjamin J. Cowling, et. al., *Viral Shedding and Clinical Illness in Naturally Acquired Influenza Virus Infections* (Journal of Infectious Diseases, https://www.ncbi.nlm.nih.gov/pmc/articles/PMC3060408/); 2010 May; 201(10): 1509–1516.

SARS-CoV-2 behaves similarly. Asymptomatic SARS-CoV-2 infected persons[132] (during the incubation period)[133] by definition are not ordinarily coughing and sneezing. Cough and sneeze cover techniques along with regular handwashing and avoiding touching one's face[134] will greatly mitigate any spread of the disease.

The notion that a person with absolutely no signs or symptoms of SARS-CoV-2 may be, in any meaningful sense, a vector of disease transmission *is simply not true.*

The peoples of the world are being subject to a *most vicious form of propaganda*: the *grossly irrational* and medically unproven idea that gargantuan SARS-CoV-2 viral replication occurs in large numbers of asymptomatic persons and is associated with high viral loads and shedding (high degree of contagion) but yet they manifest no symptoms nor observed inflammation of the nasal and pharyngeal mucosa or other areas of the respiratory tree.

With regards to Covid-19, it has been demonstrated that its severity (virulence) is generally on par with bad "flu"[135] of other

---

[132] many of whom will never develop symptoms; and this lack of symptoms correlates with low viral load and infectivity potential.

[133] defined as the time frame between onset of infection and the exhibition of symptoms, if they are to develop.

[134] It is to be noted, parenthetically, that face-masking has all but destroyed this recommendation as it has been irrefutably demonstrated that masked persons "cannot stop" touching their faces.

[135] The term "flu" is often widely misunderstood (by laypersons and health care professionals alike) to be equivalent to "influenza." SARS-CoV-2 is one of about 200 microbes (predominately viruses) that can cause flu syndromes (there are a number of non-infectious diseases that can cause "flu"—influenza-like illness). Therefore, having the "flu" describes only a

microbial causes—especially influenza. The most recent data confirms past impressions that SARS-Cov-2 is not highly contagious[136] as it is spread by droplets (person to person contact especially in a family setting) and not ultrafine aerosol (like measles[137]) and, for those in low risk groups, carries a very small, almost negligible mortality rate.

As Covid-19 is of minor consequence for most of the population, containment efforts are best directed at isolating the *KNOWN* sick and those in high risk populations. How this is to be done in the protection of higher risk populations can *ONLY* be determined by patients and their families—with the advice of his/her physician(s).

It is known by personal medical experience that many infirm and aged people fear social isolation much more than they fear any risk to themselves by an infectious agent.

To conclude this section, it is helpful to look at the actions of Jesus (as the God-Man) during His earthly life and ministry as they relate implicitly to the concept of "social distancing" when asymptomatic. The Lord Christ, as the Creator and Sovereign over *every*

---

syndrome (a collection of signs and symptoms: cough, fever, shortness of breath, muscle aches, headache, nasal congestion, etc.) but cannot inform us as to the cause of those symptoms. Testing is mandatory for accurate diagnosis. Most people with the "flu" *DO NOT* have influenza or any strain of coronavirus. See TN Department of Health data discussed earlier.

[136] Lei Luo, PhD; Dan Liu, PhD, et. al., Contact Settings and Risk for Transmission in 3410 Close Contacts of Patients With COVID-19 in Guangzhou, China, A Prospective Cohort Study (Annals of Internal Medicine, https://doi.org/10.7326/M20-2671) August 13, 2020, accessed 8/31/2020.

[137] Measles virus can even be found in the water vapor of each exhaled breath amongst the infected.

microbe in the universe, has perfect understanding of disease, pestilence, and plague. He sends and stops them and to His own glory mostly keeps them quiescent.[138]

Prior to His resurrection, Jesus had the fully human body of natural man. He bled. He became tired and hungry. He slept. He had emotions. He had daily bodily elimination functions. He had normal bacterial flora on His skin and, like modern men, probably trillions of viruses as part of His microbiome.

Plagues in the ancient World during this time were well known and relatively frequent.[139]

Given these considerations, we see in the sinless, earthly behavior of Jesus that He made no effort to "social distance" nor was there any teaching to encourage it or promote its need.

Large crowds followed Him (Luke 14:25), pressed in on him (Luke 5:1), touched Him (Mark 5:27, 31), and came to Him for healing (Luke 9:11) of a multitude of diseases, some of which were contagious as determined by the priests. He healed the mother-in-law of Peter from fever (Matthew 8:14). In a saying, He even made analogy regarding the need for human physicians, explicitly teaching that one can know when they are sick (Matthew 9:12).

Interestingly, He engaged in practices that some may consider unhygienic. He washed the certainly filthy, microbial-laden feet of

---

[138] Exodus 4:11; Deuteronomy 28:20-24.

[139] Christine A. Smith, *Plague in the Ancient World: A Study from Thucydides to Justinian* (Loyola University-New Orleans History Journal, http://people.loyno.edu/~history/journal/1996-7/Smith.html); 1996, accessed 8/31/2020.

His disciples (John 13:4-5). He allowed His feet to be kissed, bathed by tears, and then dried by a woman's hair (Luke 7:44-46). He even cured a man's blindness with spit-laden mudballs (John 9:6-7).

As Jesus kept the Law of God perfectly on behalf of His elect so they would not suffer the curses of the Covenant of Works, we dare not say that, in these actions of the sinless Christ, He failed to "do the right thing." Our Lord, by His example, did not endorse the principle of self-protection by isolation of self or others in the name of social distancing.

The Misinterpretation and Misapplication of "Love Thy Neighbor"

We have now arrived at the very crux of our discussion. If our Lord's great and vitally important commandment[140, 141] to love our neighbor is misused, serious consequences abound—not the least of which can be infringement of Christian liberty and the illicit binding of the conscience.

This principle is very broad and encompasses the six commandments[142] of the second table of the moral Law (Ten Commandments). These directives regulate how a man is to interact with his fellow men.

---

[140] Exodus 20:13, "You shall not murder," the 6th commandment.

[141] WCF LC, Q: 134-136.

[142] Honor parents, do not murder, do not commit adultery, do not steal, do not bear false witness (lie), do not covet.

The 6th commandment clearly requires of us[143, 144, 145] a duty to preserve the health, well-being, and life of those around us as much as is *feasible and rational*. However, this should not be to the point where we sinfully neglect our other duties before the Lord, which most certainly includes the gathering of His people for public worship.

All of life is a constant risk/benefit analysis, and no one but the individual or family can stand in judgment of another's level of risk tolerance. As such, men fighting in a just war in the *defense* of the nation are not in violation of the 6th commandment. Neither are Christians who drive automobiles, skydive, pilot small aircraft with passengers, work in coal mines, handle firearms, build and operate nuclear power plants, or who take care of very sick coronavirus patients in hospitals. Neither are Christians who consent to risky surgery nor those who, after considering the "costs," decline risky surgery. Christians are free to take or not take a vaccine and make either choice without coercion. Christians are not sinning should they engage in public activity with a common cold.

Christians should make every reasonable effort to avoid spreading a communicable disease. However, this concept must be considered rationally.[146]

---

[143] Primarily, individuals and families.

[144] Exodus 20:13, "You shall not murder," the 6th commandment.

[145] WCF LC, Q: 134-136.

[146] Those of us who have larger families know that some degree of respiratory contagion (especially in winter) is frequently present, especially with young children in the household.

To state the obvious, humans cannot prevent the spread of communicable diseases but merely mitigate against them; and, with respect to viral respiratory diseases, not much can be done at all. **That humans can or could have meaningfully "stopped the spread" of Covid-19 around the globe is sheer folly and should not have been attempted.** [147, 148]

In light of these considerations (and suggested by many early on in the pandemic), it was recommended that congregations assemble for worship as follows:

(a) High risk individuals should be encouraged to stay home (*but ONLY IF THEY CHOOSE to do so*).

(b) Congregants who voluntarily attend should feel well, be free of flu-like signs and symptoms (including fever), and be without *KNOWN* Covid-19 exposure (without use of appropriate personal protective equipment).

(c) Those with tender consciences[149] are to be lovingly and patiently excused.

---

[147] The only reasonable response was to, as best as possible, isolate the known sick and to make strong efforts to lessen the risks to those high-risk individuals in nursing homes and long-term care facilities and elsewhere.

[148] T.R. Allen, A.F. Bradburne, et. al., An outbreak of common colds at an Antarctic base after seventeen weeks of complete isolation (Great Britain, J. Hyg., Camb. https://www.ncbi.nlm.nih.gov/pmc/articles/PMC2130424/pdf/jhyg00082-0026.pdf); 1973. Vol. 73. Pp. 657-667, accessed 9/12/2020.

[149] In this context, defined as those uncomfortable in disregarding the edicts of the civil magistrate and/or those who consider the virus to be a significant threat to the life and health of many including themselves. Nevertheless, if such a threat is disproven or abates, a return to public worship is mandatory unless persons are *otherwise* providentially hindered.

In these recommendations, *ALL* requirements of the 6th commandment have been met. As most worshippers will be in a low risk group, Covid-19 is of little concern. As has been noted by many, exposure and infection in this population greatly enhances herd immunity (which, in turn, substantially and increasingly protects those in our families and communities with weakened immune systems).

No one's conscience has been violated. Those in high risk groups who attend public worship have done so by *their* free choice. This is also true for those who feel duty-bound to attend public worship, having determined by their own personal assessment and conscience, that they are not providentially hindered by a virus. The opinions of the civil magistrates in this decision-making are irrelevant.

What can be done about asymptomatic, potentially (but not definitively) infected persons? If a person is not sick, how can he know with certainty that he has a communicable virus? And at any given point in time, how could any non-sick person anywhere in the whole world know with inevitability they were contagious or not contagious? And when would this quandary not be true? *Of course, the answer is...NEVER.*

For millennia, Christians have regularly attended public worship during ever present and yearly "flu seasons" and until now nobody gave it much thought. All aspects of civil society have functioned normally as most people would avoid others while ill, especially if sick with fever. If persons felt well, however, they moved about freely.

Every worship service (or any public gathering for that matter) in world history has been attended by an asymptomatic person(s) who was/is potentially infected with a communicable disease. It is a "problem" for which no *rational* solution exists.

Failure to consider these important questions often ultimately causes one to engage medical absurdity *(reductio ad absurdum)* and arbitrariness.[150]

Each man must decide the risks and benefits of his actions as measured by the yardstick of God's moral law. Love for neighbor is not an emotion or sentiment but is demonstrated by an earnest desire to obey (imperfectly in this life) the commands of Christ (John 14:15; John 14:21; John 15:10). *Obedience to the moral law is love.* ***Any biblically lawful activity, such as attending church services***[151] ***when not sick, can never be declared unlawful ... by anyone.***

Another bewildering effect of the pandemic narrative has been the redefining as to what it means to be sick.

We must not tell a person that he is in sin or not "doing the right thing"[152] when he does not act as if sick when he's truly not sick. To do so is to unlawfully bind a man's conscience and is, in most cases, a violation of the 9th commandment ("you shall not bear false witness...").

---

[150] As to both, for example, the notion that the virus is a respecter of group size and won't spread if less than 11 people have gathered together.

[151] or as applied to pastors and elders, in the preaching of the Word and administration of the sacraments.

[152] "Doing the right thing" is an ethical imperative. The "right thing" can only be determined by the express or reasonably deduced demands of the moral law of God found only in Scripture.

An asymptomatic person without known recent and direct contact with a contagious person cannot know, in any ordinary sense, that he is or is not afflicted with a transmittable disease. A man is not responsible before God for that which he *CANNOT* know.

Clerical Decisions to Suspend Public Worship During the Pandemic Were Built on Faulty Premises [153]

Faulty Premise Number One

The discipline of biblical apologetics and its methods are not relevant to the Covid-19 account. A multitude of ecclesiastical leaders largely abandoned the application of a Christian world and life view to the Covid-19 pandemic narrative. This necessarily led many to explicitly engage Faulty Premise Two.

---

[153] Not all church councils fell prey to all, some, or even any of the defective presuppositions enumerated herein. Even when they did, it was often subconsciously held. Some churches briefly closed simply given the mass confusion and hysteria manifest during the early days of the pandemic lock-downs. In essence, the decision was made to shut down, gather wits, "take a deep breath," research, and try and figure out "what's going on here!?" We have little quibble with these church leaders and their decision-making processes. In many cases, these were the last congregations to suspend normative church activities and the first to re-open.

Faulty Premise Number Two

The belief that the mainstream Covid-19 narrative is true, a priori. Christians are commanded to be "salt and light" in the world[154] and to "expose the darkness" wherever it is to be found.[155] This requires discernment and a search for truth in all of life. Given that what was offered in the Covid narrative was a spiritually dark, high stakes venture,[156] a prompt and vigorous search for the truth by all in Christ's church should have promptly commenced.

Faulty Premise Number Three

The idea that the duties of local church governments include the specifics of medical analysis, interpretation of medical data, and subsequent decision making on behalf of their congregants. This came about as a result of failing to consider what Scripture teaches church officers regarding *the primary* duty and the *boundaries* of their authority—the watching over the *souls* of the flock (Hebrews 13:17). Minding the souls of the flock does not include the duty or authority to ordinarily

---

[154] Matthew 5:13-16.

[155] Ephesians 5:11.

[156] In the U.S., it is now apparent that the devastating economic consequences of "our response" and the corresponding loss of civil liberties will *MASSIVELY* dwarf anything the virus was/is capable of doing. "Better safe than sorry" is not rooted in a biblical world view. If we are required to "count the cost" in our following of Christ, we are required to do so in other earthly endeavors (an argument from the greater to the lesser [Luke 14:28-33]).

concern themselves with the general health and safety of the congregation in any primary or preventative sense.

Of course, the elders are to make reasonable efforts to secure the safety of the congregants *during public* worship and other uses of *church property* (e.g. fire exits, avoidance of fire hazards, property maintenance, church security, and in strongly encouraging the contagious *sick* to stay home amongst other reasonable and rational courses of action).

But the day to day health and safety risks of the individual and family are *outside of the elders' domain*. What congregants eat, what medical treatments they take, whether or not they exercise, what vaccines they take or do not take, and whatever decisions they make regarding the risk tolerances of their various life activities are *NOT* within the province of church councils *unless* an activity be clearly shown to be *forbidden* or, if not being performed, *required* by the Word of God. *Otherwise, to interfere in these matters is to bind the consciences of the congregants.*

Prior to the disruptions of Covid-19, ordinary *personal* providential hindrances to public worship were easily identified and typically agreed upon.[157] *Corporate* hindrances to worship are typically

---

[157] *Personal:* illness; out of town and without reasonable access to a faithful Christian church; transportation difficulties; ice/snow storms; works of necessity and mercy on the Lord's Day and the like; *Corporate:* The majority or even all of the elders of the church are dead, missing, or incapacitated by illness or injury; ice and/or snow storms and other severe, dangerous weather events that may reasonably and imminently occur during the time of assemblage; floods and other causes of impassable roads, earthquakes and war; sudden inhabitability of the church building, etc.

extraordinary and usually of brief (day to day, week to week, not months or indefinite) duration.

Interestingly, the yearly influenza pandemics have *NEVER* caused the widespread suspension of public worship services across the nation. The mere presence of "flu season" was never considered a de facto reason to suspend corporate worship. In the United States, smallpox was endemic well into the early 20th century; church gatherings were not ordinarily suspended merely because disease outbreaks existed somewhere.

As it has been conclusively established that Covid-19 risks for the vast majority of congregants are lower than that of influenza, the churches should not have closed as a result of the novel coronavirus pandemic *as it never rose to the level of a legitimate, extraordinary providential hindrance to gathering.*

Faulty Premise Number Four

That church officers were necessarily beholden to the Covid-19 diktats of the civil magistrates and public health officers. This notion has been thoroughly refuted earlier in the chapter. As established, the civil magistrate has no ecclesiastical authority. Period.

The concept that the magistrate possess unlimited quarantine powers is an egregious error that unwittingly aids and abets the possibility of tyranny in broader civil society which certainly will affect the Christian Church. As part of their prophetic ministry to the civil magistrates, the church is to proclaim to them their godly duty to protect the church and be "nursing fathers and mothers" to her (Isaiah 49:23; WCF 23.3*).[158]

Faulty Premise Number Five

That church councils possess the duty and authority to decide for their congregants as to what the membership should think about Covid-19 and its narrative and to then impose this narrative upon them. It is readily apparent that a multitude of opinions abound in and outside of the Church regarding all facets of the Covid-19 chronicle. In this context, *the only wise* course for the elders was and is to *let Christian liberty reign.*

It is truly incomprehensible that church officers would take it upon themselves to define and interpret SARS-CoV-2 for Covid-19 dissenting congregants under their charge, whether a physician or non-physician. From a Presbyterian perspective, this represents a form of ecclesiastical absolutism[159] and is to be roundly condemned.

---

[158] "... Yet, as nursing fathers, it is the duty of civil magistrates to protect the Church of our common Lord, without giving the preference to any denomination of Christians above the rest, in such a manner that all ecclesiastical persons whatever shall enjoy the full, free, and unquestioned liberty of discharging every part of their sacred functions, without violence or danger."

[159] "We are the church officers, we have ruled, so it shall be."

Faulty Premise Number Six

That church officers had the right and duty (ostensibly to protect health) to bind the consciences[160, 161] *of those asymptomatic congregants who, based on their own assessment of the situation,*[162] *concluded that they were not providentially hindered by Covid-19 from attending to the public worship of God.* This is most serious, as gathering for corporate worship is *a* if not *the* foundational duty of Christ's visible church and is explicitly commanded in the Word of God. These actions also violate the spirit of 1 Peter 5:3:

...not domineering over those in your charge, but being examples to the flock.

---

[160] In most cases, this was mostly done unwittingly and subconsciously and with no intended malice. Nevertheless, the unwarranted hindering of access to public worship and all that it entails is an egregious error.

[161] PCA *BCO*; II. 1. and 7; pp. 10-11: (1) "God alone is Lord of the conscience and has left it free from any doctrines or commandments of men (a) which are in any respect contrary to the Word of God, or (b) which, in regard to matters of faith and worship, are not governed by the Word of God. Therefore, the rights of private judgment in all matters that respect religion are universal and inalienable." (7) "All church power, whether exercised by the body in general, or by representation, is only ministerial and declarative since the Holy Scriptures are the only rule of faith and practice. No church judicatory may make laws to bind the conscience. All church courts may err through human frailty, yet it rests upon them to uphold the laws of Scripture though this obligation be lodged with fallible men."

[162] and conducted in Christian liberty.

The authors, two of whom are physicians, never at any time felt that SARS-CoV-2 was a providential hindrance to themselves in any medical or ecclesiastical sense. We were not ill, had no transportation difficulties, and no Lord's Day works of mercy and necessity that prevented us from presenting ourselves, with our families, for the corporate worship of God. Pastors and ruling elders were readily available, and the church buildings were deemed structurally safe for occupancy. Yet, because of a fairly ordinary virus (one that is survived by about 99.8% of those infected), we were indeed deprived admittance to the in-person public preaching of the Word and the administration of the sacraments as well as other accompaniments of congregational life.

How did the Bible-believing, conservative, and evangelical churches arrive at the point by which the sheep had to earnestly contend and plead with their Shepherds to allow them access to public, corporate worship?

Conclusions to Biblical Limitations of Ecclesiastical Power

1. The government of the church does not derive its authority from the state but from Christ and Christ alone.
2. The government of the church is distinct from the civil magistrate and, in ecclesiastical matters, answerable *only* to God by way of His Law-Word.

3. The civil magistrate has no ecclesiastical authority whatsoever and may not interfere with any aspect of church government, most especially any decisions regarding congregational assembly.

4. The courts of the church have *no primary duty* related to congregational health and safety. The *CHIEF* responsibility for health and safety resides in and with the individual and family.

5. The foundational duty of the elders is to "watch over the souls" of the congregants in their charge, primarily by the reading, preaching and teaching of the Word, administration of the Sacraments, prayer, and church discipline as well as other prescribed forms of worship.

6. In the suspension of corporate public worship, a multitude of congregations often failed to ask important questions: Is the narrative true? Is it to be believed a priori? Does the civil magistrate have authority to govern worship? Do the church elders possess unlimited authority?

7. The Covid-19 pandemic narrative and the sundry responses to it are beset by a multitude of medical, epidemiological, and theological problems.

8. It was mistakenly held that church officers possessed the duty and authority to (a) impose upon the consciences of their congregants as to what they are to believe regarding the pandemic narrative[163]

---

[163] That the narrative was true (despite much evidence in opposition to it) and that SARS-CoV-2 represented a serious threat to the health and life of almost everyone despite the contrary testimony of their own observations and experiences and other medical and theological data points.

and (b) use that imposition to bind the consciences of those healthy congregants who in their rejection of the mainstream Covid-19 account did not feel providentially hindered from public worship. Nonetheless, they were barred indeed from church entry for a time without Scriptural warrant. This was despite the fact that these individuals willingly shouldered all responsibility for their own risk tolerance of SARS-CoV-2 infection.

9. Lastly, by the sanctifying power of the Holy Spirit, may the Church strive vigorously to grow in grace as a consequence of the lessons learned from the pandemic and (a) evermore be "salt and light" to the world and labor continuously to "expose the darkness" wherever it may be found; (b) endeavor always to "count the cost" in all of our decision making for the sake of Christ; (c) be increasingly discerning; and (d) not be in imitation of the world (as ones living without Christ and without hope) in times of trouble and, particularly, to strenuously avoid living in doubt and fear as Christ is always with us.[164]

---

[164] *What is your only comfort in life and in death?* --- Question One: Heidelberg Catechism (1563):

That I, with body and soul, both in life and in death,[1] am not my own,[2] but belong to my faithful Savior Jesus Christ,[3] who with His precious blood[4] has fully satisfied for all my sins,[5] and redeemed me from all the power of the devil;[6] and so preserves me[7] that without the will of my Father in heaven not a hair can fall from my head;[8] indeed, that all things must work together for my salvation.[9] Wherefore, by His Holy Spirit, He also assures me of eternal life,[10] and makes me heartily willing and ready from now on to live unto Him.[11]

[1]Rom. 14:7-8. [2]I Cor. 6:19. [3]I Cor. 3:23. [4]I Pet. 1:18-19. [5]I Jn. 1:7; 2:2. [6]I Jn. 3:8. [7]Jn. 6:39. [8]Mt. 10:29-30; Lk. 21:18. [9]Rom. 8:28. [10]II Cor. 1:21-22; Eph. 1:13-14; Rom. 8:16. [11]Rom. 8:1.

May all Believers often dwell on these extraordinary principles. Amen!

CHAPTER 5

A Cure Worse than the Disease

Joel E. Yeager, MD

In a late March news conference, President Trump stated, "We cannot let the cure be worse than the problem itself."[1] This well-known aphorism of a cure worse than the disease is attributed to the English philosopher and statesman Francis Bacon who warned of a "remedy worse than the disease."[2] Since we chose to keep our office open during the pandemic, I started hearing multiple stories which highlighted exactly that. By late April I had already heard versions of the following stories.

- Farmers were pouring thousands of gallons of milk down the drain or into the manure pit, despite empty store shelves.[3]

---

[1] We've all heard this countless times since the President made this comment on Monday, March 25, 2020. (See https://www.foxnews.com/media/cure-worse-than-disease-trump-pundits-would-ease-virus-restrictions, accessed 9/8/2020.)

[2] Bacon (1561-1626) ended an essay entitled "Of Seditions" where he warned that if princes did not maintain good relationships with the military as well as other "great men in the state; or else the remedy, is worse than the disease." (See http://www.authorama.com/essays-of-francis-bacon-16.htmlm accessed 9/8/2020.)

[3] Some have suggested this was because workers were "too sick" to show up at processing plants. Perhaps that was the case in some communities. I think it was largely due to shutdowns and fear as discussed in previous chapters.

- Chicken farmers gassed entire flocks of chickens and hog farmers slaughtered entire houses.
- Beef farmers struggled from low beef prices.
- Fifty trucks at a local trucking company sat idle, losing tens of thousands of dollars in revenue.
- Construction crews were unable to work, even though there may have only been several men on the crew and working outside! No job meant no money.
- *I have numbness and tingling in both of my arms when I lay down at night. I'm not sure if it's my asthma or my anxiety.*
- A young patient who had finally recovered from a severe case of trichotillomania (hair-pulling) now has bald patches again.
- Elective surgical procedures were placed on hold, so I treated a toe with an anti-inflammatory, knowing the patient would need an injection two weeks later.
- *Things were finally looking up after 5 years of bad milk prices. I made some financial commitments as a result, and now I'm not sure.*

These scenarios have been multiplied exponentially throughout the country over the past months. The term *iatrogenic* in medicine essentially means "we caused it." Throughout this chapter, I will explore four iatrogenicides[4] resulting from Covid-19—medical,

---

[4] *Iatrogenic* is a poor medical outcome caused by us, the physicians. I'm using *iatrogenicide* to mean a "death caused by us" (us being society in general). While not necessarily actual deaths, each of these categories represent a trend which leads toward death rather than life in the broad sense.

emotional, economic, and spiritual "cures" all far worse than the disease itself.

A Professional Betrayal

I have been reading the works of C.S. Lewis this year. Sometime in late May I read these haunting words from *The Abolition of Man*:

> The final stage [of Man's conquest of Nature] is come when Man by eugenics, by pre-natal conditioning, and by an education and propaganda based on a perfect applied psychology, has obtained full control over himself. *Human* nature will be the last part of Nature to surrender to Man. The battle will then be won...But who, precisely, will have won it?

> For the power of Man to make himself what he pleases means, as we have seen, the power of some men to make other men what *they* please...the man-moulders of the new age will be armed with the powers of an omnicompetent state and an irresistible scientific technique: we shall get at last a race of conditioners who really can cut out all posterity in what shape they please.

> The Conditioners, then, are to choose what kind of artificial *Tao* [what Lewis defines as Natural Law or Traditional Morality] they will, for their own good reasons, produce in the Human race.

...Thus at first they may look upon themselves as servants and guardians of humanity and conceive that they have a "duty" to do it "good"...They recognize the concept of duty as the result of certain processes which they can now control...They know quite well how to produce a dozen different conceptions of good in us. The question is which, if any, they should produce...

...But I am not supposing [the Conditioners] to be bad men. They are, rather, not men (in the old sense) at all. They are, if you like, men who have sacrificed their own share in traditional humanity in order to devote themselves to the task of deciding what "Humanity" shall henceforth mean...

...It is not that they are bad men. They are not men at all. Stepping outside the *Tao*, they have stepped into the void. Nor are their subjects necessarily unhappy men. They are not men at all: they are artefacts. Man's final conquest has proved to be the abolition of Man [underlined emphases mine].[5]

When I read this section in Lewis earlier this year, I realized he was describing our current society, and specifically the betrayal I felt as a medical professional being spoon-fed information that I knew didn't pass the muster of scientific scrutiny. What I never fully understood

---

[5] Lewis, C.S. (1943, 1946, 1978). *The Abolition of Man*. London: Fount, An Imprint of HarperCollins Publishers, pp. 36-40. This was given by Lewis as the Riddell Memorial Lectures (Fifteenth Series) at the University of Durham, February 1943.

Lewis to mean by "men without chests" I now realized was right in front of me. Lewis wrote that "the head [what he called *cerebral* man] rules the belly [what he called *visceral* man] through the chest—the seat...of emotions organized by trained habit into stable sentiments... It may even be said that it is by this middle element [the Chest] that man is man: for by his intellect he is mere spirit and by his appetite mere animal."[6] The function of a society described above is to produce "Men without Chests."[7] Unfortunately, is that not what we see in much of our Covid society? **"Chestless" pawns (society) who are subservient to the Conditioners (government and science), who act as an "omnicompetent state" using an "irresistible scientific technique" comprised of "education and propaganda based on a perfect[ly] applied psychology" to obtain "full control" over society?** And who has been responsible for this masquerading charade? My own medical profession, who as pointed out elsewhere in this volume, had to know better!

Let me highlight this professional betrayal with several examples. *First*, despite the overwhelming evidence against masks presented elsewhere in this volume, masked mandates remain the *tour de force* of church, school, business, medical, and other policies.

My emotions range between humor and anger when I see a single masked driver in an enclosed vehicle with windows up! Or while seated outdoors at a restaurant and fellow diners at an adjacent table

---

[6] Ibid, p. 15.
[7] Ibid.

have masks on until dinner is served.[8] Or when I read of choir policies which limit rehearsal times to 30 minutes, distances between choir members of ten feet, and masks on except when singing. I would like to believe C. S. Lewis when he wrote that our neighbors are "a society of possible gods and goddesses" and that we "have never talked to a mere mortal."[9] Yet I can't help but realize that a deceptive lunacy has fallen over society like a shroud, snuffing out light, truth, and free-thinking.[10] Why?

Physicians and public health departments have hidden behind "a growing body of evidence" which supposedly supports the use of face masks and human interventions which allow us to control the virus at will. Rancourt[11] has forcibly critiqued this supposed evidence.[12]

---

[8] My wife and I observed this at one of our favorite local restaurants on 9/11/2020. It is fair to assume that gathering friends from different families were not wearing masks at home and arrived to dinner without masks. (The latter was an observed fact as we were seated outdoors at the entrance to the restaurant and I observed no masked diners arriving via vehicle to the restaurant.) Yet masks were put on when different friends arrived at the same table and removed when dinner was served. What changed?!

[9] Lewis, C.S. (1949, 1962, 1965, 1975, 1980). *The Weight of Glory and Other Addresses.* (W. Hooper, Ed.) New York: Simon & Schuster, p. 39. Lewis is writing about the dignity of humanity and goes on to say, "But it is immortals whom we joke with, work with, marry, snub, and exploit—immortal horrors or everlasting splendors."

[10] I can only hope and pray that this is a prequel to the motto of the Protestant Reformation, *post tenebras lux* (after darkness, light).

[11] Rancourt is referenced in footnote #77 in chapter 2.

[12] Rancourt, D.. (2020). Face masks, lies, damn lies, and public health officials: "A growing body of evidence". DOI: 10.13140/RG.2.2.25042.58569. This was published on August 3, 2020 and is available online at the listed DOI. Several pages of this report outline his scientific credentials, including his research supervision at the doctoral level, 100+ peer-reviewed

212

He states that the "growing body of evidence" is a "vile new mantra" which serves as a "propagandistic phrase" designed to achieve five main goals:

1. Give the false impression that a balance of evidence now proves that masks reduce the transmission of COVID-19.
2. Falsely assimilate commentary made in scientific venues with "evidence."
3. Hide the fact that a decade's worth of policy-grade evidence proves the opposite: that masks are ineffective with viral respiratory diseases.
4. Hide the fact that there is now direct observational proof that cloth masks do not prevent exhalation of clouds of suspended aerosol particles; above, below and through the masks.
5. Deter attention away from the considerable known harms and risks due to face masks, applied to entire populations.[13]

Rancourt points out a key betrayal by the medical community in ignoring the gold-standard of evidence—the randomized controlled trial (RCT)—in favor of observational or cohort studies.[14] "Thus, we

---

scientific publications, and greater than 5,000 citations in peer-reviewed journals. While physicians are trained in science, I heartily concur with his statement: "It would be insufficient for me to be a simple medical doctor (MD) or public health officer"! I highly recommend reviewing the entire 36-page PDF document.

[13] Ibid, pp. 1-2. These five points are bulleted in the original. I have numbered them for emphasis.

[14] See, for example, Wang Y, Tian H, Zhang L, et al Reduction of secondary transmission of SARS-CoV-2 in households by face mask use, disinfection and social distancing: a cohort study in Beijing, China. *BMJ Global Health* 2020;5:e002794. This "provides the first

see that the WHO and local public health officials are hindering advancement, by promoting non-RCT 'observational studies', rather than protecting public health."[15] He further states:

> It should be of great concern to all that the WHO pretext of "a growing compendium of observational evidence on the use of masks by the general public in several countries"[16] has morphed into the mantra "a growing body of evidence", which finds itself on the lips of virtually all public health officers and city mayors in the country.

> This mantra of "a growing body of evidence" is advanced as the false silver bullet justification for draconian masking laws, in actual circumstances in which:

---

evidence of the effectiveness of mask use…" This is a *cohort* and not an RCT study and typical of the type of evidence used by pro-maskers. Rancourt (p. 19) cites "the world's leading medical standards and medical statistician expert," Dr. Janus Christian Jakobsen, who states: "Clinical experience or observational studies should never be used as the sole basis for assessment of intervention efforts—randomized clinical trials are always needed." (See "The Necessity of Randomized Clinical Trials", by Jakobsen and Gluud, in the British Journal of Medicine & Medical Research. 3(4): 1453-1468, 2013.) Rancourt further points out that 1) non-RCT studies of the antiarrhythmic drugs flecainide and encainide were very promising when the drugs went to market until an RCT showed they increased mortality and 2) decades of non-RCT observational studies were the basis for HRT's (hormone replacement therapy) reported decrease in heart attacks until published RCTs in 2002 showed they actually *increased both* heart attacks *and* breast cancer (p. 21).

[15] Ibid, p. 5.

[16] This is from page 6 of WHO's "Advice on the use of masks in the context of COVID-19: Interim guidance," 5 June 2020. WHO Reference Number: WHO/2019-nCov/IPC_Masks/2020.4, available online via reference number.

➤ There have been NO new RCT studies that support masking

➤ All the many past RCT studies conclusively do not support masking

➤ None of the known harms of masking have been studied (re: enforcement on the entire general population).

This is the opposite of science-based policy. The politicians and public health officers are actuating the worst decisional model that can be applied in a rational and democratic society: forced preventative measures without a scientific basis while recklessly ignoring consequences.

In this article, I prove that there is no policy-grade evidence to support forced masking on the general population, and that all the latest decade's policy-grade evidence points to the opposite: NOT recommending forced masking on the general population.

Therefore, the politicians and health authorities are acting without legitimacy and recklessly.[17]

While rather technical, the contrast described above between the non-RCT versus the RCT trial is *critical to understanding the*

---

[17] Rancourt (source in footnote #11), pp. 5-6. The "expert opinions" cited in the "growing body of evidence" are often modelling studies, op-ed style opinions, population studies, overview reports, etc., and "all are susceptible to large bias." See p. 28.

professional betrayal by medicine and the scientific community. This is not to say that non-RCT trials have no place in science; they certainly do, and I've cited some in my review. The point is, however, that research validated over years by the gold standard of clinical research (the RCT) is now being displaced and even discarded by less stringent standards. Rancourt further notes a Tweet by the medical officer of Toronto Public Health stating that "there is a growing body of emerging evidence that shows that non-medical masks can help prevent the spread of COVID-19." Rancourt states:

> This is squarely false. There is not a single published scientific study "that shows that non-medical masks can prevent the spread of COVID-19", let alone "a growing body". In order to measure "the spread of COVID-19", one has to actually measure "the spread of COVID-19". In fact, there is a growing body solely of spin and of false statements about the scientific research literature [emphasis added; punctuation as used by author].[18]

All of us have *seen* this spin. Unfortunately, many have not recognized it *as* spin. In my state of Pennsylvania, federal coronavirus money had been withheld by our Governor to our own Lebanon County because our local elected officials had pushed back against our Governor's harsh lockdown measures. The $13M was finally released, but with the stipulation that $2.8M of it needed to go to a mask

---

[18] Ibid, p. 18.

education campaign. Shortly thereafter, notices from our Department of Health started including all the above narrative, publicly shaming those people who choose not to wear a mask. This professional betrayal of actual science has been parroted by churches and parachurch organizations who have now ventured into the role of public health officer. This is evidenced on church web sites outlining masked mandates and reasons for the same, seminaries following the mantra for return to class, and places like The Ethics and Religious Liberty Commission of the Southern Baptist Convention in an article entitled "Explainer: How masks can help prevent the spread of COVID-19."[19]

Good science and expert evaluation should always look at the complete picture. The first rule of medicine dating to Hippocrates is *primum non nocere*, or "first, do no harm."[20] Yet strangely lacking in

---

[19] See https://erlc.com/resource-library/articles/explainer-how-masks-can-help-prevent-the-spread-of-covid-19/, published July 24, 2020, accessed on this date when it arrived via email. In my opinion, one of the most egregious affronts to truth in this article is this statement: "If 95% of Americans wore face masks in public, it could prevent more than 45,000 deaths by Nov. 1, according to the University of Washington's Institute for Health Metrics and Evaluation." On the surface, this sounds impressive and a moral imperative couched in "how Jesus would certainly have responded in love and self-effacement" (my paraphrase) seems unarguable. However, as Rancourt has pointed out above, there is no RCT (nor will there ever be) that has ever confirmed this. All such predictions are computer-generated mathematical probability studies, which while interesting are essentially useless in terms of truth. It troubles me that Christians can't sort this out. However, my profession is responsible for perpetrating this iatrogenicide and the church has simply parroted it.

[20] It is my duty as a physician to make certain that what I recommend to my patients first causes no harm. This is sometimes referred to ethically as *nonmaleficence*. This is followed by a second ethical principle of *beneficence* or causing good. I discuss these two principles with patients quite frequently.

the "growing body of evidence" is the analysis of potential harm done by universal masking.[21] Consider these examples (in no particular order):

1. *Mask mouth*

   "Meth mouth" describes poor oral hygiene associated with chronic meth users. Dentists are now recognizing something similar in "mask mouth," which is chronic gum inflammation associated with constant mask-wearing. "Gum disease—or periodontal disease—will eventually lead to strokes and an increased risk of heart attacks," according to Dr. Marc Sclafani, dentist and co-founder of One Manhattan Dental. A colleague at the same dental practice reported that 50% of his patients were suffering negative health effects from chronic mask-wearing. People tend to breathe through their mouth

---

[21] Another alarming trend in the "growing body of evidence" mantra is discarding previous information. Since March 2020, I've kept a rather extensive file of articles and videos on Covid. It's interesting to see some of those articles now removed, and not just on social media. For example, I had saved an article by a dentist entitled "Why Face Masks Don't Work: A Revealing Review," by John Hardie, BDS, MSc, PhD, FRCDC. (All those letters mean he's a dentist with a Master of Science and a PhD who is a Fellow of The Royal College of Dentists of Canada. In other words, not your average dentist!) I originally accessed that article on 6/14/2020. Today (9/12/2020), I re-accessed it and was met with this demeaning comment: "If you are looking for 'Why Face Masks Don't Work: A Revealing Review' by John Hardie, BDS, MSc, PhD, FRCDC, it has been removed. The content was published in 2016 and is no longer relevant in our current climate." (See https://www.oralhealthgroup.com/features/face-masks-dont-work-revealing-review/.) Whoa! Just like that. Some editor made that sweeping assertion, and what I recall was a well-articulated article is gone. *That should be shocking to anyone interested in free speech and enquiry.*

rather than nose while wearing a mask, contributing to dry mouth, decrease in saliva, and bacterial overgrowth contributing to dental caries.[22]

2. *Mask contamination*

One doctor has described masks as "basically a giant Petri dish you have strapped to your face."[23] Is that true? Doctors and nurses (158 participants) from fever clinics and respiratory wards in three hospitals in Beijing, China between December 2017 and January 2018 allowed their medical masks to be evaluated after their shifts. Viruses were found in 10.1% of the masks, including adenovirus, bocavirus, respiratory syncytial virus, and influenza virus. The positive virus rate was 14.1% in masks worn for greater than 6 hours and 16.9% in those who examined greater than 25 patients per day. 83.8% reported at least one problem with mask wearing, including facial pressure, difficulty breathing, discomfort, trouble communicating with the patient, and headache.[24]

---

[22] As reported in the *Washington Examiner* on August 7, 2020, available at https://www.washingtonexaminer.com/news/mask-mouth-dentists-warn-prolonged-use-of-masks-leading-to-poor-oral-hygiene, accessed 9/12/2020. My wife introduced me to this term while reading another news article about a month ago.

[23] From https://nofacemask.blogspot.com/2020/05/doctor-says-face-mask-is-basically.html, accessed 9/12/2020.

[24] Chughtai, A.A., Stelzer-Braid, S., Rawlinson, W. *et al*. Contamination by respiratory viruses on outer surface of medical masks used by hospital healthcare workers. *BMC Infect Dis* 19, 491 (2019). https://doi.org/10.1186/s12879-019-4109-x.

One of England's most senior doctors and deputy chief medical officer, Dr. Jenny Harries, told the BBC News that masks can "actually trap the virus" and "for the average member of the public walking down a street, it is not a good idea."[25]

Rancourt points out that home fabric masks are *hydrophilic* whereas medical masks are *hydrophobic*.[26] To translate, cloth masks "like" water while medical masks don't! In other words, cloth masks absorb water and medical masks repel it. He points out that this difference hasn't been studied or mentioned. You don't really need to be much of a scientist to know that damp, moist environments are "breeding grounds" for pathogens! Or as one of my patients stated in common sense vernacular, "Would you hook up your exhaust pipe to your intake?!"

3. *Acne mechanica, aka "maskne"*

    I was introduced to this by my niece who works as an RN in a university hospital. According to Nazanin Saedi, board-certified dermatologist at Thomas Jefferson University, "maskne is acne formed in areas due to friction, pressure, stretching,

[25] As reported in the *Independent*, March 12, 2020, at https://www.independent.co.uk/news/health/coronavirus-news-face-masks-increase-risk-infection-doctor-jenny-harries-a9396811.html, accessed 9/12/2020.

[26] Rancourt, Face masks…, p. 15.

rubbing or occlusion. You can see it in the areas covered by the mask and also the areas where the mask and face shields touch the skin." It is triggered when skin pores are blocked by sweat, oil, and makeup due to friction. Breathing for extended periods of time with masks on creates lots of humidity which is "a breeding ground for acne."[27]

4. *Respiratory problems & decreased immunity*

    "Fact-checkers" almost always debunk the claim that mask-wearing inhibits oxygen flow. Vernon Coleman, MB, ChB, DSc, FRSA, is a British international best-selling physician-author and medical critic. In one of his "bloke in a chair" videos, he states:

    > …so, the wearing of masks will in my view result in far more deaths than could possibly be saved. Wearing a mask reduces blood oxygen levels…There will, before long, be a disaster with a bus crashing because the driver was wearing a mask and became hypoxic. Why else do you think governments everywhere admit that people with respiratory or heart problems don't have to wear a mask? That's proof—if ever it was needed—that these things affect oxygen levels.[28]

---

[27] As reported on https://www.health.com/condition/skin-conditions/maskne-mask-acne-mechanica, accessed 9/12/2020.

[28] My transcript from his video, available at https://www.youtube.com/watch?v=u047hrU5osw&feature=youtu.be, accessed ~9/5/2020.

A study of the blood oxygen levels of 53 surgeons before and after surgeries revealed a decrease in blood oxygen levels post-surgery which was directly correlated to the duration of mask-wearing.[29] Neurosurgeon and nutritional expert Dr. Russell Blaylock notes that this decrease in oxygen levels—otherwise known as hypoxia—is critical because it "is associated with an impairment in immunity. Studies have shown that hypoxia can inhibit the type of main immune cells used to fight viral infections called the CD4+ T-lymphocyte…This sets the stage for contracting any infection, including COVID-19 and making the consequences of that infection much graver. In essence, your mask may very well put you at an increased risk of infections and if so, having a much worse outcome."[30] Blaylock further notes that mask-wearing will prevent viruses from being exhaled, allowing for concentration in the nasal passages and entrance to the brain via the olfactory nerve.[31]

---

[29] Beder A, Büyükkoçak U, Sabuncuoğlu H, Keskil ZA, Keskil S. Preliminary report on surgical mask induced deoxygenation during major surgery. *Neurocirugia (Astur)*. 2008;19(2):121-126. doi:10.1016/s1130-1473(08)70235-5. During the week of this editing (early October 2020), "new studies" are being published showing that masks have absolutely no effect on oxygen levels, including those with COPD! Do I smell a rat?!

[30] See https://www.technocracy.news/blaylock-face-masks-pose-serious-risks-to-the-healthy/?fbclid=IwAR2fnRrdw-F4_wGaDPoeZ_NVyD_IzU6LZ8YkDug-MyDtZ7PKF0irucc2o9es, accessed 9/12/2020.

[31] Perlman S, Jacobsen G, Afifi A. Spread of a neurotropic murine coronavirus into the CNS via the trigeminal and olfactory nerves. *Virology*. 1989;170(2):556-560. doi:10.1016/0042-6822(89)90446-7. This demonstrated that a mouse coronavirus entered the brain by way of the olfactory and trigeminal cranial nerves.

5. *Others*

128 out of 158 (81%) healthcare workers in Singapore "developed de novo PPE-associated headaches."[32] Vision difficulties occur due to fogging of glasses. Communication is extremely hindered through a face mask as one cannot see facial expressions.

A *second* form of professional betrayal is in the inaccurate testing for Covid as well as the false reporting of Covid deaths, both reviewed by Dr. O'Roark in the previous chapter.

Third, the rush to a vaccine appears to me to be a form of professional betrayal. While I am not opposed to the development of a Covid-19 vaccine per se, I do not believe that the "best way to get this virus under control is through a universal vaccine."[33] That sounds heretical coming from a physician; let me explain.

Vaccines are most effective when they target diseases which only reside in one host—in this case humans. Take smallpox as an example of a human disease which has been successfully eradicated. (We don't vaccinate against it anymore because it no longer exists.) It used to be a highly visible and distinct disease and it also only affected humans. Contrast that with yellow fever, which can affect humans but

---

[32] Ong JJY, Bharatendu C, Goh Y, et al. Headaches Associated With Personal Protective Equipment - A Cross-Sectional Study Among Frontline Healthcare Workers During COVID-19. *Headache.* 2020;60(5):864-877. doi:10.1111/head.13811.

[33] This is not a direct quote, but it is part of the mantra and narrative with which we are constantly bombarded.

also animals such as monkeys. "If a mosquito capable of spreading yellow fever bites an infected monkey, the mosquito can then give the disease to humans. So even if the entire population of the planet could somehow be vaccinated against yellow fever, it's eradication could not be guaranteed."[34]

Coronaviruses come from a very large family of viruses known as *Coronaviridae*. The genus *alphacoronavirus* is known to affect pigs, cats, dogs, humans, and bats. The genus *betacoronavirus* affects humans, cattle, pigs, antelope, giraffes, mice, humans, rats, and bats; MERS and SARS are in this genus. *Gammacoronavirus* affects chickens, turkeys, and whales while *deltacoronavirus* affects birds and pigs.[35]

SARS "originated from horseshoe bats in China as its animal reservoir and transmitted to humans after amplification in palm civets from wildlife markets," while "dromedary camels in the Middle East are the immediate animal source of the MERS epidemic caused by MERS coronavirus (MERS-CoV)."[36] Viruses mutate (change) all the

---

[34] From "The History of Vaccines: An Educational Resource by the College of Physicians of Philadelphia," available at https://www.historyofvaccines.org/content/articles/disease-eradication, accessed 9/13/2020.

[35] See the American Veterinary Medical Association at https://www.avma.org/sites/default/files/2020-02/AVMA-Detailed-Coronoavirus-Taxonomy-2020-02-03.pdf, accessed 9/13/2020.

[36] Susanna K.P. Lau, Antonio C.P. Wong, Libao Zhang, Hayes K.H. Luk, Jamie S. L. Kwok, Syed S. Ahmed, Jian-Piao Cai, Pyrear S.H. Zhao, Jade L.L. Teng, Stephen K.W. Tsui, Kwok-Yung Yuen, Patrick C. Y. Woo. Novel bat alphacoronaviruses in southern China support Chinese horseshoe bats as an important reservoir for potential novel coronaviruses. *Viruses*. 2019 May; 11(5): 423. Published online 2019 May 7. doi: 10.3390/v11050423.

time and there appears to be crossover among the coronavirus family members. "Bats are the reservoir of a wide variety of coronaviruses, including severe acute respiratory syndrome coronavirus (SARS-CoV)-like viruses. SARS-CoV-2 may originate from bats <u>or unknown intermediate hosts</u> and cross the species barrier into humans [emphasis added]."[37]

Professor Ian Frazer is a clinical immunologist trained in Scotland and professor at the University of Queensland in Australia as well as an elected Fellow for the Royal Society in London (2012). He is the co-inventor of the technology which enabled the HPV vaccine.[38] He argues that coronaviruses have been hard historically to make vaccines for because they infect the upper respiratory tract, "which our immune system isn't great at protecting" and which makes it a difficult target area for a vaccine. He states:

"It's a separate immune system, if you like, which isn't easily accessible by vaccine technology."

"It's a bit like trying to get a vaccine to kill a virus on the surface of your skin."

"One of the problems with corona viruses [sic] in the past has been that when the immune response does cross over to

---

[37] Guo YR, Cao QD, Hong ZS, et al. The origin, transmission and clinical therapies on coronavirus disease 2019 (COVID-19) outbreak - an update on the status. *Mil Med Res*. 2020;7(1):11. Published 2020 Mar 13. doi:10.1186/s40779-020-00240-0, from Figure 1.

[38] See his bio at The University of Queensland Australia at https://researchers.uq.edu.au/researcher/228, accessed 9/13/2020.

where the virus-infected cells are it actually <u>increases the pathology rather than reducing it</u>...So that immunisation [sic] with SARS corona vaccine <u>caused, in animals, inflammation in the lungs which wouldn't otherwise have been there if the vaccine hadn't been given</u> [emphases added]."[39]

According to the World Economic Forum, vaccine development typically occurs through five stages over a course of ten years at a cost of up to $500 million.[40] Those five stages look like this:

1. Discovery research (2 to 5 years)
2. Pre-clinical trials (2 years, which often includes animal experimentation and possibly less than 15 humans); these first two are sometimes referred to as Phase 0.
3. Clinical development
   a. Phase I (1-2 years), involving 20 to 80 people, asks *is it safe?*
   b. Phase II (2-3 years), involving several hundred people, asks *does it activate an immune response?*
   c. Phase III (2-4 years), involving several thousand people, asks *does it protect against the disease?*
4. Regulatory review and approval (1 to 2 years)

---

[39] From https://www.abc.net.au/news/health/2020-04-17/coronavirus-vaccine-ian-frazer/12146616, accessed 9/13/2020.

[40] From https://www.weforum.org/agenda/2020/06/vaccine-development-barriers-coronavirus/, accessed 9/13/2020.

5. Manufacturing and delivery (often referred to as Phase IV, or post-marketing surveillance).[41]

If you do the above math, you don't really get to Phase III until around year 7. Yet Dr. Fauci announced that Moderna began its Covid-19 Phase 3[42] trials involving 30,000 patients in early July.[43] Moderna itself announced on May 29, 2020 that it was enrolling 600 patients in its Phase 2 study.[44] So Phase 3 was underway about the same time Phase 2 was just getting started! While it's true that the FDA granted Moderna "Fast Track" designation, one can only imagine what corners are being cut in such a rush to vaccine development.

The push for a vaccine also flies in the face of an emerging trend in medicine, particularly the idea that early exposure to something[45] may heighten the body's immune response and thereby prevent an adverse response. It's the basis of what our parents told us often—*a little dirt never hurt anyone!* An article in *The New England Journal of Medicine* several years ago[46] evaluated asthma risk in Amish and Hutterite farm children. This was of interest to me since I practice

---

[41] See also https://www.healthline.com/health/clinical-trial-phases, accessed 9/13/2020. This is the standard process for any drug or vaccine development.

[42] Arabic and Roman numerals are used interchangeably in referring to trials.

[43] See https://www.forbes.com/sites/brucejapsen/2020/06/02/fauci-modernas-phase-3-covid-19-vaccine-trial-will-include-30000-young-and-old-individuals/#32a391e54f75, accessed 9/13/2020.

[44] See https://investors.modernatx.com/news-releases/news-release-details/moderna-announces-first-participants-each-age-cohort-dosed-phase, accessed 9/13/2020.

[45] Usually referred to in medicine as an *antigen*.

[46] I downloaded this article the same day of its publication date, 8/4/2016.

among the Amish. Amish utilize traditional farming as opposed to Hutterites who utilize industrial farming. Even though the Amish farms were clean, the close proximity of houses and barns "indicate that the Amish environment provides protection against asthma by engaging and shaping the innate immune response."[47] In other words, they didn't develop asthma because they were exposed to controlled dust from little up.

Shortly after that, one of my patients asked me about "peanut paste" for young children. The preceding dictum was that peanuts should be avoided in children before age three because of the risk of a severe allergic reaction known as anaphylaxis. While this was new to me, it followed in the steps of the *NEJM* article above, in that "even children with the highest risk of having a peanut allergy should be tested with a tiny dose of peanut, because it might prevent the allergy from ever developing"![48]

So our bodies are able to take care of themselves under the right circumstances? Absolutely! Yet here we have a universal push for a vaccine when our bodies are generally able to handle this virus on their own. As Dr. Blaylock notes,

---

[47] M M Stein et al. Innate Immunity and Asthma Risk in Amish and Hutterite Farm Children. *N Engl J Med* 2016; 375:411-421; DOI: 10.1056/NEJMoa1508749.

[48] See https://www.today.com/health/peanut-allergies-prevent-them-little-peanut-t106706, published 1/5/2017, accessed 9/13/2020. The article quotes Dr. Matthew Greenhawt, allergist at Children's Hospital of Colorado: "We actually want all children to have peanut introduced" by age 6 months.

The fact that this virus is a relatively benign infection for the vast majority of the population and that most of the at-risk group also survive, from an infectious disease and epidemiological standpoint, by letting the virus spread through the healthier population we will reach a herd immunity level rather quickly that will end this pandemic quickly and prevent a return next winter. During this time, we need to protect the at-risk population by avoiding close contact, boosting their immunity with compounds that boost cellular immunity and in general, care for them.[49]

Lockdowns and isolation tend to increase inflammatory responses throughout the body (generally a bad thing). I first heard this described by Dr. Shiva Ayyadurai, PhD in a recorded video interview, where he states: "The two most disastrous things are that we're socially distancing people and hiding them. Go look at the research...when you isolate people, that is one of the worst [contributors] to obesity, smoking, and heart disease. Social isolation actually leads to upregulation of inflammatory compounds in the body and downregulation of antiviral compounds. So you're basically increasing the person['s risk] for viral infection by the amount of stress you're causing them from social isolation..."[50] They also tend to *decrease* rather than increase our

---

[49] See footnote #29.

[50] My own transcript of the video interview available at https://www.youtube.com/watch?v=86VJlhw0DQQ. I originally encountered this video in early June 2020, but later in my research was "surprised" to find that it had been removed. I was able to find and access again on 9/13/2020. Of course, Wikipedia [with no documentation] describes him as a "promoter of conspiracy theories and unfounded medical claims"!

immune systems (also a bad thing). There appears to be protective cross-reactivity between previous human coronaviruses (HCoVs) and SARS-CoV-2.

> ...prior immunity induced by one HCoV has also been reported to reduce the transmission of homologous and, importantly, heterologous HCoVs, and to ameliorate the symptoms where transmission is not prevented. A possible modification of COVID-19 severity by prior HCoV infection might account for the age distribution of COVID-19 susceptibility, where higher HCoV infection rate in children than in adults, correlates with relative protection from COVID-19, and might also shape seasonal and geographical patterns of transmission.
>
> Public health measures intended to prevent the spread of SARS-CoV-2 will also prevent the spread of and, consequently, maintenance of herd immunity to HCoVs, particularly in children. It is, therefore, imperative that any effect, positive or negative, of pre-existing HCoV-elicited immunity on the natural course of SARS-CoV-2 infection is fully delineated.[51]

The explanation of this PhD from MIT appeared entirely scientific to me, so one can only wonder as to the reason for the unfounded Wikipedia claim!

[51] Kevin W. Ng et al. Pre-existing and *de novo* humoral immunity to SARS-CoV-2 in humans. bioRxiv 2020.05.14.095414; doi: https://doi.org/10.1101/2020.05.14.095414, posted 7/23/2020, preprint. This positive and protective cross-reactivity explains why I personally felt mild Covid-19 symptoms occurring at least 6 or 7 times over the past few months, only to wake up the next morning entirely fine. LuAnne and I (like all PCPs) have been exposed

The conservative commentator Daniel Horowitz writes in his commentary on this study:

> In other words, don't mess with God's natural design, especially when fewer kids die from this than from the flu. Not only will endless distancing of children playing together harm kids, but it forecloses on the best shot of achieving herd immunity with the lowest-risk population, thereby shielding the more vulnerable. Imagine how many other viruses will now percolate longer in society and endanger the vulnerable because we've tampered with God's intelligent immunological ecosystem and prevented kids from passing it around.[52, 53]

Based on my clinical experience, I predict that this push for a vaccine over and above our own innate immunity will inadvertently add fuel to the already-growing fire of anti-vaccination sentiment. Add to that a rather horrifying discovery I made in the vaccine trial literature, and with that we transition to the second *emotional* iatrogenicide.

---

to hundreds if not thousands of upper respiratory viruses over the course of our clinical careers. It would therefore be entirely unnecessary for us to receive the Covid vaccine.

[52] From https://www.theblaze.com/conservative-review/horowitz-lockdown-children-harming-immune-systems-best-shot-herd-immunity, published 7/28/2020, accessed 9/13/2020.

[53] Less than a week before this manuscript went to print, three professors from Harvard, Oxford, and Stanford met in Great Barrington, Massachusetts and formulated the Great Barrington Declaration on October 4, 2020 (available at www.gbdeclaration.org, accessed 10/6/2020). It calls for the healthy to return to normal to develop herd immunity.

Shamed into Compliance and Driven to Despair

The Lancet reports that "one advantage of universal use of face masks is that it prevents discrimination of individuals who wear masks when unwell because everybody is wearing a mask."[54] Wrap your head around that statement! In yet another subversive twist, the modus operandi of "masked mandaters" seems to be to shame people into wearing masks. The *"Wear a mask. Protect others"* lingo which appears at the top of current CDC websites on Covid-19 and that I critiqued in chapter two certainly operates on the premise of shaming non-maskers into submission with the overt assumption that not wearing a mask means you're not interested in others—or even worse, that you're interested in killing others.[55]

While police stand hamstrung in cities awash in the tinder and ash of rioting violence, employees in stores across the country have become the "masked patrol" who not-so-subtly enforce mask wearing on its patrons. Those who choose not to wear masks receive announcements via overhead speakers that "all customers are reminded to wear masks while in store." Senior pastors are given the job of communicating elder board decisions to parishioners, all the while ignoring those whose consciences disallow participation in said charade. What seems to be the underlying theme in all of this? *We will shame*

---

[54] See reference source in footnote #60, chapter 2.

[55] Watch any social media video of current riot protestors across our country and you'll hear this language used routinely.

you into complicity. And our society, from physicians to senior executives, has become extremely complicit in the national narrative.

Is this happenstance, as in everyone just *happens* to be saying the same thing? What if, in fact, we've all been primed, as Tom Nikkola suggests?[56] What if phrases such as the CDC reminder above or *we're all in this together* or *stay safe, stay home* are 21st-century examples of behavioral priming? What if the goal is to teach society that "those who don't follow the conventional recommendations aren't in this with you"? Or to show that they're "outsiders" and such are "easy to target and hate and slander," as Nikkola writes? After all, "behavioral priming can lead us to believe something is a fact even without evidence to support it. It would explain why some people feel it's okay to throw stones at those who believe in something other than staying home. They want to slander doctors who suggest we're actually safer being at work."[57]

In the horrifying discovery I alluded to above, I found just such behavioral priming overtly stated. In the "COVID-19 Vaccine Messaging, Part 1" website of the U.S. National Library of Medicine, 4,000 participants in a vaccine trial will be randomized to 10 treatment arms (and 2 control arms) assessing the participants willingness to receive a COVID-19 vaccine within 3 and 6 months of it becoming

---

[56] See Tom Nikkola, "What if we've all been primed?" at https://tomnikkola.com/prime/?fbclid=IwAR3IcOCfF6NmWCPF2vNu-ALSo9QUzwJzKGTHZumgjE0MYhsYAIw9S8mspL0c, accessed 5/14/2020, re-accessed 9/13/2020.

[57] Ibid.

available.[58] The ten treatment arms for this Covid-19 vaccine study include the following messaging:

- *Personal freedom message* – "COVID-19 is limiting people's personal freedom and by working together to get enough people vaccinated society can preserve its personal freedom."
- *Economic freedom message* – "[same language as above]...by working together...society can preserve its economic freedom."
- *Self-interest message* – "COVID-19 presents a real danger to one's health, even if one is young and healthy. Getting vaccinated...is the best way to prevent oneself from getting sick."
- *Community interest message* – "...a message about the dangers of COVID-19 to the health of loved ones. The more people get vaccinated..., the lower the risk that one's loved ones will get sick..."
- *Economic benefit message* – "...COVID-19 is wreaking havoc on the economy and the only way to strengthen the economy is to work together to get enough people vaccinated."
- *Guilt message* – "...asks the participant to imagine the guilt they will feel if they don't get vaccinated and spread the disease."

---

[58] Review at https://clinicaltrials.gov/ct2/show/study/NCT04460703?term=Vaccine&cond=Covid19&cntry=US&draw=2, accessed 8/7/2020, re-accessed 9/13/2020.

- *Embarrassment message* – "...asks the participant to imagine the embarrassment they will feel if they don't get vaccinated and spread the disease."
- *Anger message* – "...asks the participant to imagine the anger they will feel if they don't get vaccinated and spread the disease."
- *Trust in science message* – "...vaccination is backed by science. If one doesn't get vaccinated that means that one doesn't understand how infections are spread or who ignores science."
- *Not bravery message* – "...describes how firefighters, doctors, and front line medical workers are brave. Those who choose not to get vaccinated against COVID-19 are not brave."[59]

Who *doesn't* see an obvious agenda in these pre-vaccine messaging trials? I can only imagine the frustration honest thinkers would feel being subjected to such *brainwashing* and *propaganda*. However, I can also imagine the messaging having its intended effect in a large portion of society who hasn't had the background we've presented here. So yes, we *are* being primed. It's right there for the record at Clinical-Trials.gov.

In addition to the very unbiblical concept of shaming,[60] the emotional tolls of Covid-19 have been widely reported and

---

[59] Ibid. To be clear, these are direct quotations from the messaging participants will receive in the clinical trial.

[60] *Shame* is always a result of the Devil as opposed to *sorrow* which is the response of the believer, as in "godly sorrow worketh repentance to salvation" (2 Corinthians 7:10, KJV).

documented. Seniors have been isolated in long-term care facilities or sick family members in hospitals often without the interaction of family and friends. Even seniors living in their own homes have been isolated from family. A meta-analysis of studies led by Dr. Julianne Holt-Lunstad, professor of psychology and neuroscience at Brigham Young University, found that lack of meaningful social interactions can raise health risks by as much as smoking 15 cigarettes per day or abusing alcohol.[61]

Gunnell et al wrote, "The likely adverse effects of the pandemic on people with mental illness, and on population mental health in general, might be exacerbated by fear, self-isolation, and physical distancing [emphasis added]."[62] As of August, the National Alliance on Mental Illness HelpLine saw a 65 percent increase in calls and emails since March.[63] The Disaster Distress Helpline at the Substance Abuse and Mental Health Services Administration saw an 891% increase in calls and text messages in March 2020 compared to March

---

[61] Holt-Lunstad J, Smith TB, Baker M, Harris T, Stephenson D. Loneliness and Social Isolation as Risk Factors for Mortality: A Meta-Analytic Review. *Perspectives on Psychological Science*. 2015;10(2):227-237. doi:10.1177/1745691614568352, as reported at https://www.engadget.com/2020-03-27-pyschological-impact-covid-19-isolation.html, accessed 9/13/2020. I only had access to the abstract of this original review.

[62] Gunnell et al. Suicide risk and prevention during the COVID-19 pandemic. *The Lancet Psychiatry*, ISSN: 2215-0366, Vol: 7, Issue: 6, Page: 468-471, published online 4/21/2020, in print 6/2020, https://doi.org/10.1016/S2215-0366(20)30171-1. Gunnell is an English epidemiologist and suicidologist at the University of Bristol.

[63] See https://www.rollcall.com/2020/08/05/pandemics-effect-on-already-rising-suicide-rates-heightens-worry/, accessed 9/13/2020.

2019.[64] Sandro Galea, MD, from the Boston University School of Public Health wrote in *JAMA Internal Medicine*, "...large-scale disasters...are almost always accompanied by increases in depression, post-traumatic stress disorder (PTSD), substance abuse disorder, a broad range of other mental and behavioral disorders, domestic violence, and child abuse."[65] He and his colleagues note the unfortunate correlation between school closings and increased child abuse.

According to the American Medical Association, "more than 40 states have reported increases in opioid-related mortality as well as ongoing concerns for those with a mental illness or substance abuse disorder."[66]

But beyond shamed, forceful complicity and a driven despair lies a third iatrogenicide of massive *economic* proportions.

Down the Tube

The economic consequences of Covid-19 are probably the easiest to see. Arbitrary government designations of "essential" versus "non-essential" businesses demeaned the biblical concept of work as described by Dr. O'Roark in chapter 4. Since the average American's

---

[64] See https://abcnews.go.com/Politics/calls-us-helpline-jump-891-white-house-warned/story?id=70010113, accessed 9/13/2020.

[65] Galea S, Merchant RM, Lurie N. The Mental Health Consequences of COVID-19 and Physical Distancing: The Need for Prevention and Early Intervention. *JAMA Intern Med.* 2020;180(6):817–818. doi:10.1001/jamainternmed.2020.1562.

[66] See https://www.ama-assn.org/system/files/2020-09/issue-brief-increases-in-opioid-related-overdose.pdf, updated 9/8/2020, accessed 9/13/2020.

job exists to put bread on the table and a roof over the family head, *any* job to the worker is essential, regardless of the job. Calling one's job "unessential" stratifies society into categories God never intended. It's true that some people "boomed" while others "busted" and the economics of Covid will likely be studied for decades to come.

In America, we saw historic low unemployment rates disappear almost overnight. We saw businesses shuttered and streets eerily silent. We heard stories of desperation as noted in the vignettes in the beginning of this chapter. Because we smelled a rat in early April, we attempted to offer a reasonable counter-perspective to the massive shutdowns occurring in our state and across the country. As noted in chapter 2, I wrote a letter to our Governor in late April. LuAnne and I wrote an extended letter to our church Session[67] in late May. We were among over 1200 signatories of a letter to President Trump calling the shutdown equivalent to "a mass casualty event."[68] I and approximately 100 other physicians participated in a video Second Opinion Project over Memorial Day weekend, telling the stories of patients harmed by government intrusion and lockdown.[69] We were

---

[67] As noted elsewhere in this volume, this is Presbyterian terminology for an "elder board."

[68] Letter available at https://disrn.com/news/mass-casualty-incident-600-doctors-sign-letter-to-trump-calling-for-end-to-coronavirus-lockdowns/; our signatures are on page 10. (The initial 600 signatures eventually doubled.)

[69] Available at https://www.secondopinionproject.com/sign39610500; my interview is available at
https://www.youtube.com/watch?v=qYNuA52GgK8&list=PL2nXC6uo9WW77yGl2zpYkpC8db0plaefc&index=11&t=0s or via YouTube search under the title "Second Opinion Project: LOCKDOWN—The cost to farmers."

also part of a letter urging President Trump to revise the onerous CDC guidelines for school reopening, which culminated in Jenny Beth Martin from the Tea Party Patriots discussing this letter with President Trump, the First Lady, and Vice President Pence at the White House on July 7. We did these things because we were and are convinced that the "cure" has been worse than the disease. The effects of our efforts remain unknown.

The obvious ill effect of this iatrogenicide needs only several substantiating facts:

- Unemployment rose from a record low of 3.5 million in February to 14.7 million in April.[70]
- Hospitals cancelled elective surgeries and procedures, causing hospitals to lose exponential amounts of money. For example, Illinois estimated that cancellations and delays were costing their hospitals alone $1.4 billion per month, according to the American Hospital Association (AHA).[71]
- The four-month loss to American hospitals and health systems between March 1, 2020 and June 30, 2020 amounts to

---

[70] See https://tradingeconomics.com/united-states/unemployment-rate, accessed 9/13/2020. The good news is it consistently fell since April and was 8.4 million in August 2020.
[71] See https://www.webmd.com/lung/news/20200506/covid-19-leaves-us-hospitals-in-financial-crisis#2, accessed 9/13/2020.

$202.6 billion, or an average of $50.7 billion per month, according to the AHA.[72]

- The average American's 401(k) and IRA were down by 19% and 14% respectively at the end of first quarter 2020.[73]

But loss of care is not only measured in economic terms. Writing in the *NEJM*, Dr. Lisa Rosenbaum recounts multiple stories of cancer and cardiac care not being given in deference to Covid-19. She quotes an interventional cardiologist at Jamaica Hospital Medical Center and Lenox Hill Hospital in New York who said, "I think the toll on non-Covid patients will be much greater than Covid deaths." Michael Grossbard, chief of hematology at New York University's Langone Hospital stated, "Our practice of medicine has changed more in 1 week than in my previous 28 years combined." She recounts the story of a 70s-year old woman with cardiac risk factors presenting to an ED with chest pressure and shortness of breath. She required urgent intubation. Chest x-ray revealed bilateral interstitial pneumonia, so she was transferred to ICU as a "Covid rule-out." While waiting for her Covid results, her troponins continue to rise. When Covid results came back negative, she underwent angiography, but by then she had developed cardiogenic shock due to coronary occlusion and

---

[72] See https://www.aha.org/guidesreports/2020-05-05-hospitals-and-health-systems-face-unprecedented-financial-pressures-due, accessed 9/13/2020.

[73] See https://www.fool.com/investing/2020/04/28/heres-the-impact-of-covid-19-on-the-average-americ.aspx, accessed 9/13/2020.

died—all because doctors focused on Covid-19 and missed the fact that she had a heart attack.[74]

As we conclude this chapter, we turn to the *fourth* iatrogenicide, which is the toll this has taken on the spiritual fabric of our churches.

The Slippery Slope

In my contribution to this volume thus far, I have primarily relied on medical and scientific data. While one of my caveats in chapter two was that I write from a biblical worldview, I have not highlighted much of that worldview up to this point. That has been intentional. This section is a fitting conclusion to this booklet, as it brings us full circle back to where we started. Why *did* the church cancel worship, and why do we as authors believe as the subtitle states that a sacred trust has been broken?

Both 2 Kings 18 and Isaiah 36 record the Assyrian king Sennacherib's invasion of Judah, using a high-ranking military officer called the Rabshakeh as his spokesman. The Rabshakeh, an enemy of God's people, asks King Hezekiah, "*On what do you rest this trust of yours? Do you think that mere words are strategy and power for war? In whom do you now trust...?*"[75] Can't you hear the sneer in his voice?

---

[74] Rosenbaum, L, The Untold Toll—The Pandemic's Effects on Patients without Covid-19, *N Engl J Med* 2020; 382:2368-2371; DOI: 10.1056/NEJMms2009984, published online 4/17/2020, in print 6/11/2020.

[75] 2 Kings 18:19-20 & Isaiah 36:4-5, ESV. My daily devotional reading happened to be from Isaiah the morning of this writing (9/13/2020)!

Do you really think this God of yours is stronger than the might of the Assyrian army?! Imagine now that the Rabshakeh is a public health officer or perhaps the Surgeon General or maybe a governor. Imagine one of them asking a pastor or a church Session or an elder board, "In whom do you now trust? Do you really believe this Providential God of yours is going to spare you from the coronavirus?!"

It grieves me to see church leadership placing their trust in CDC and Department of Health guidelines over and above the sovereignty of God. It grieves me to see churches bow to the behavioral priming of media narratives and dress it up in the biblical language of love, humility, and community witness—all the while conveniently ignoring truth offered to them as alternatives. It grieves me to see majority opinions ruling when inconvenient truths and minority voices are conveniently dismissed. It grieves me to see churches and parachurch organizations run de facto by Dr. Fauci rather than by a stated trust in God's sovereignty. I've heard senior pastors tell congregations that this will soon all be a blip in the rearview mirror when things are back to normal. I believe the stakes are far higher than that, and that this brief blip represents an epoch when good men failed and chose the easy route by obeying men rather than God.

On the bright side, I've never heard so often how much the leadership loves the church! On a slightly darker side, I've also tired of hearing church leadership exhort their congregations to "be safe." Since when has safety become the modus operandi of the church? As Dr. O'Roark has pointed out, it really isn't the church's business to ensure our safety. I'm reminded of Lucy asking Mr. and Mrs. Beaver in *The Lion, The Witch and the Wardrobe* whether Aslan was safe.

> "Safe?" said Mr. Beaver; "don't you hear what Mrs. Beaver tells you? Who said anything about safe? 'Course he isn't safe. But he's good. He's the King, I tell you."[76]

But, you say, there's so many opinions that it's hard to tell who to believe. Unfortunately, this has become a convenient excuse to ignore inconvenient truths and a reason not to engage with alternatives. We have attempted in this small volume to present cogent facts within the framework of a Christian worldview. We have cited multiple medical and scientific authorities. These are not our opinions. But beyond these facts is the larger question the church has failed to answer—*how do you determine truth and on what do you base that conclusion?* And herein lies the rub. This has *never* been an issue of opinion for myself, my wife and physician partner, nor my two author colleagues. This has *always* been a matter of truth. This is why I cannot in good conscience participate in church functions which dance a choreographed script of mask-on-for-this-mask-off-for-that illusion.[77] As I have pointed out elsewhere, these restrictions on based on two <u>false</u>

---

[76] Lewis, C.S. (1998?), *The Complete Chronicles of Narnia*, Collins, An Imprint of Harper-Collins Publishers, p. 99. (This book doesn't have a publication year, but it was purchased in England over the centennial of Lewis' birth in 1898. It has delightful "illustrations hand-coloured by the artist, Pauline Baynes.")

[77] Examples of this would be masks on while walking in a church hallway but off in a classroom or masks on while not singing in a rehearsal but off while singing.

illusions—that masks work and that we are all asymptomatic spreaders of Covid.

If church leaders resort to the "that's your opinion" narrative, then the church is guilty as charged for operating from a postmodern mindset where truth is true based on one's preference of truth.[78] For if the church cannot sort out truth on something like coronavirus, what guarantees do parishioners have that they'll speak truth on bigger issues?

Permit me to quote from my wife in an email at the end of May:

> All of us have faced the "threat" of picking up virus droplets from others all our lives – from the tender moments the whole family comes to see a newborn baby to singing in school Christmas programs to holding hands while saying grace around the dinner table to visiting Grandpa in the hospital after his surgery! We have never gone to church or baseball games or grocery shopping or family gatherings without a very real "threat" of picking up a germ. And we are all healthier today because we *did* pick up germs and have developed immunity through getting ill.
>
> COVID-19 is nothing different. Our greatest protection against this "invisible enemy" is our God-given immune

---

[78] Nancy Pelosi famously illustrated this when she told the Department of Homeland Security Secretary Kirsten Nielsen, "I reject your facts." To which Nielsen replied, "These are not my facts. These are the facts." See https://www.redstate.com/elizabeth-vaughn/2019/01/05/pelosi-dhs-secretary-kirsten-nielsen-reject-facts/, accessed 9/13/2020.

systems. Trusting in masks and measuring tapes rather than trusting in the amazing ability of our immune systems comes awfully close to blasphemy—which Webster defines as *the act of insulting or showing contempt...for God.* Is that too harsh? Our Father has protected all of us from dying from viruses many, many times! (Literally every single viral infection we get has the potential to trigger our demise—just like COVID-19 does.) Somehow the church as a whole is buying into mass hysteria over this pandemic, focusing on *fearmongering* by the media and the *protocols for control* established by the medical establishment. Why is God and Truth getting a back burner this time around? Just because this is medical? I'm sorry, but just because we doctors have protocols and treatment algorithms for everything doesn't mean we are powerful enough to "control outcomes" the way all our medical journals like to suggest. Joel and I see this deceptive assumption being swallowed hook, line, and sinker by the church in our response to this "crisis."[79]

Let me offer some final challenges. What would our persecuted brothers and sisters say about our safety and social distancing? Those brothers and sisters risk life and limb and walk for hours just to get inside a church. What would they say?

What would the Romans have said about the modern American church? Would we be "guilty as charged" by Pliny the Younger in his *Letters to Trajan?*

---

[79] From an email written by LuAnne D. Yeager, MD, dated 5/28/2020.

They affirmed, however, the whole of their guilt; or their error, was, that they were in the habit of meeting on a certain fixed day before it was light, when they sang in alternate verses a hymn to Christ as to a god, and bound themselves by a solemn oath, not to do any wicked deeds, but never to commit any fraud, theft or adultery, never falsify their word, nor deny a trust when they should be called upon to deliver it up...[80]

Tabor further notes that the Romans saw the Christians "as spreading like a <u>contagious disease</u> among the naïve and foolish classes [emphasis added]."

What if *the church* is being primed? What if coronavirus was a test to see what Christians really believe? What if a supposed public health crisis was the first stop on the slippery slope continuum? What if Christians are declared by government the "contagious disease" of our generation because we teach a life and sexual ethic out of step with the cultural milieu? What if we are declared a public health threat? Will our complicity with a perceived public health threat guarantee our complicity with the next? That next step on the slippery slope is far closer than we think.

So, in *whom do you now trust?* And *on what do you rest this trust of yours?* Our current context highlights the somber reality of those

---

[80] As noted in a column by James D. Tabor, Professor of Religious Studies at University of North Carolina at Charlotte, entitled "The Christians as the Romans Saw Them: Superstitious, Depraved, Obstinate, and Foolish," available at https://www.huffpost.com/entry/the-christians-as-the-rom_b_4037301, accessed 6/21/2020, re-accessed 9/13/2020.

words. They should lead us all to repentance. They should lead us all to our knees. They should lead us all to the foot of the Cross. For it is there that our perspectives are reoriented, and it is there that we realize that "God has not given us a spirt of fear, but of power and of love and of a sound mind" (2 Timothy 1:7, NKJV).

Soli Deo Gloria!

CONCLUSION

The Way Forward is the Way Home

> "Give unto the LORD the glory due
> unto his name; worship the LORD
> in the beauty of holiness."
> Psalm 29:2 (KJV)

Much now has expounded upon this subject of closing the house of God due to the coronavirus, and sadly we must conclude that the majority who did so were resting upon weak and unsound principles. As we have thought about the matter of cessation of the public gathering of God's people for worship and the position of most in the Evangelical and Reformed community, clearly church leadership has the popular national—if not international—majority on its side in its position. *Then again, truth is not found in a popularity contest.* But what emanates forth so obviously by most who argue for that majority position, is that it is one of human consideration, medical collaboration, community opinion, peer coordination, and government cooperation. Yet what seems to be missing is direct, clear, and conclusive biblical support for ecclesiastical interruption. With ill-advised yet declarative decrees, Romans 1:22 rings forth, "*Professing themselves to be wise, they became fools.*" As Christians we want to be guided by the Scriptures in every step, and as Reformed and Presbyterian believers, we want to be directed and governed by the Standards the church professes to follow. We do not see either in the cessation of public worship activity. As members of a Reformed and Presbyterian Church, we feel we are not being shepherded and guided biblically, but rather have a sense of being corralled and confined. What a strange irony to witness the members of a church pleading with their shepherds in defense of public gathering for worship in God's House.

The position that so many churches had taken to suspend public worship and lock out the people of God has had serious divisive consequences for the visible Church. It is bringing about a sifting of those who are faithful to God in wanting public worship versus those who trust in the arm of flesh and man. It will serve to have even worse results if these orders continue, or should a future wave of virus occur and church leaders enact another shutdown. **This must never happen again**!

It is important to ask: *how may the church immunize herself against future extraordinary shutdowns?* The answer is as noted in Chapter 4 and worth repeating here:

> *Scripture (as the ultimate and final authority), the Westminster Standards, biblical law, a proper presuppositional apologetic method, an exegetically sufficient understanding of biblical church-state relations, use of biblically wholesome man-made civil laws, and a Christian world and life view that self-consciously informs medical, scientific, and statistical* (we would add here civil, familial, and ecclesiastical) *methodologies.*

Christians must ask the following questions regarding the diktats of others (inquiries which are vitally applicable to all areas of life):
What *is* the authority (Scripture)? Who *has* authority (Jurisdictionalism)? Are the "dictators" trustworthy (biblical apologetics)? Is the un-
derling paradigm true and even knowable (biblical epistemology)? Is
the request "lawful" (biblical law)? Have we been salt and light? Have
we exposed the darkness? Have we counted the cost? Have we avoided
ungodly fear and anxiety? Have we honored Christ in all things by
striving in all our endeavors to glorify Christ?

The way home is usually traveled by "old paths." One doesn't
get home by seeking out new paths. While the intelligent believer will
always be open to new understandings, these can never replace or su-
persede well-established old paths, and "new normals" which defy old
paths must never be allowed to take root in church, medical, or social
culture. So, what is the way home medically? It's quite simple—*if
you're sick or vulnerable, stay home. If you're not, return to pre-Covid nor-
malcy.* All the best science is on the side of these old paths.

Your Only Comfort in Life and In Death

The Heidelberg Catechism is justly regarded as one of the fin-
est summaries of the Christian faith ever written. First published in
1563, the catechism is used by more than a million Christians globally.
The first question of the catechism is among the most beloved of the
Reformed confessions and catechisms:

Q. 1. *What is thy only comfort in life and death?*

A. *That I with body and soul, both in life and death, am not my own, but belong unto my faithful Savior Jesus Christ; who, with His precious blood, hath fully satisfied for all my sins, and delivered me from all the power of the devil;* **and so preserves me that without the will of my heavenly Father, not a hair can fall from my head;** *yea, that all things must be subservient to my salvation, and therefore, by His Holy Spirit, He also assures me of eternal life, and makes me sincerely willing and ready, henceforth, to live unto Him* [emphasis added].

The emphasis here is to highlight the total confidence and security we have in God in the face of disease and death. This is not a blind trust, or some reckless disregard for medical science or a denial of using the brain given us by the Creator. Rather, it is an affirmation of the belief and expectation that places full assurance in our Savior with a knowledge that He desires our regular praise, honor, and worship as the corporate and covenant family of believers.

Is not this your life of joy in the Lord? Doesn't this encourage in you a thrill at the expectation of the next Lord's Day gathering where God will meet with His people? Are you not hungering and thirsting for the righteousness of hearing the Word of God read and preached in the Sanctuary of meeting? Do you not delight with rightful excitement out of gratitude to hear what the Lord God Almighty will speak to your heart through His servant in the pulpit?

In a post by R. Scott Clark entitled, *"Your Only Comfort in Life and In Death,"* Clark explains the background to this first catechism question and particularly the matter of our hope and trust in troubling times—times not just "like a plague" but in fact during an actual plague. He says:

> *This question and answer was not written in a vacuum. Medieval life, which includes the 16th century, the period in which the Reformation began, was not an easy time in which to live... When the authors and editors of the Heidelberg Catechism asked about the Christian's comfort 'in life and in death' it was not a mere theory. Death was a frequent visitor to Heidelberg and to every pre-Modern city. Tuberculosis was widespread. Caspar Olevianus (1536–87), one of the principals behind the catechism died of it. The plague came to Heidelberg and took many lives... In 1566 Heidelberg itself, was afflicted with the plague. Even though most fled, including the court, Olevianus, who was the chief pastor, and Zacharias Ursinus (1534–83) stayed behind to minister to plague victims.... We are Christians. We are a purchased people. Covid-19 is not the Black Plague— which some survived. We know that this world is not random. The Savior who purchased us by his obedience and death will not abandon us. Should he will to take us out of this life, we will go to be with him who loves us. This is not to be cavalier but to try to put our fears into some perspective. The world tells us that this*

life is all there is. So, they panic. By contrast, we make prepara-
tions.[1]

So, we challenge church leadership to trust in the Lord and
"Give unto the Lord the glory due unto his name: bring an offering, and
come before him: worship the Lord in the beauty of holiness." (1 Chronicles
16:29). Make your leadership ready as one who heeds the call of service to God and let your hearts *"Serve the Lord with gladness: come be-*
fore his presence with singing." (Psalm 100:2). This has only been one
test for your faithfulness. So often in the Bible we are called to "remember" an event, the work of God, and yes, to remember our own
sin and shortcomings. More tests will follow. Will we be mindful of
our response to the current crisis? The Church of Jesus Christ is under
assault, as evidenced in society's disdain and government overreach.
The level of overt hostility and manifest control will bring trials and
terrors to the hearts of men of truth. The increase of hatred for those
who profess faith in Christ is almost eschatological in appearance. But
as Psalm 124:8 says, *"Our help is in the name of the LORD, who made*
heaven and earth." Amidst all that comes upon us, you as leaders, for
the sake of the flock, must not waiver, nor acquiesce to the wisdom of
worldly solution and compromise. The Scripture is paramount to your
decisions. The actions you take must first and foremost be with a
mind's eye for obedience to the commands of God, whereby your true
love for the Savior is demonstrated. Your shepherding care, exercised

---

[1] https://heidelblog.net/2020/03/your-only-comfort-in-life-and-in-death/, accessed
8/19/2020.

in the church, should "*do good unto all men, especially unto them who are of the household of faith*" (Galatians 6:10).

Hope for the future is not without promise. The Lord blesses His Church, and where it falters, the way forward is the way home, and the way home is the way of hope, and the way of hope is the way of confession and repentance, for it brings the Church closer to the One who is merciful, full of compassion, long-suffering, and who affords forgiveness. We cannot simply move on without a remediated communion with GOD. In our Lord is comfort and peace through a faithful walk of life that trusts His Sovereign Will and gracious hand of love and care through our Savior Jesus Christ. May we all move onward with the words of Psalm 122:1 upon our lips saying, "*I was glad when they said unto me, Let us go into the house of the Lord.*"

Ernest Springer, III
Joel E. Yeager, MD
Daniel O'Roark, DO, FACC

...ask for the old paths... Jeremiah 6:16

Old Paths Publications was established as a ministry for the cause of Christ and His Church. We seek to offer timely titles for the purpose of edification and instruction.

In our day, where true Christianity is increasingly under attack, *Old Paths Publications* endeavors to bring together a united and confessional Reformed and Presbyterian thought, through the publishing of Gospel truths given to us by the Spirit of God through His faithful elect, as they saw the fast approaching storm of Apostasy.

It is our hope and prayer that we may be of service to you, that our books might ring true to the Word of God, and that the Lord Jesus Christ might be exalted by all for His own glory.